The Visual Guide to Swedish Massage

The Visual Guide to

Swedish
Massage

Mark F. Beck

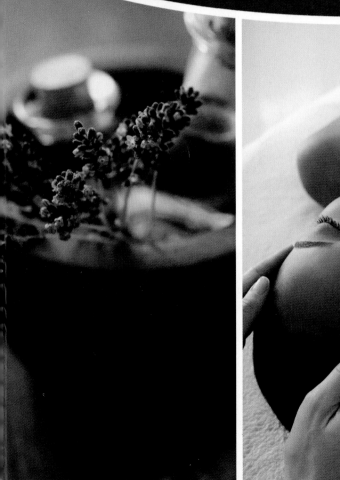
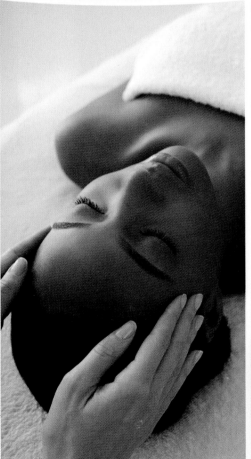
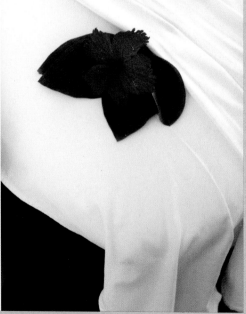

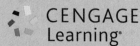

CENGAGE
Learning

Australia • Brazil • Japan • Korea • Mexico • Singapore • Spain • United Kingdom • United States

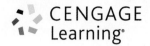

The Visual Guide to Swedish Massage
Mark F. Beck

Vice President, Milady & Learning Solutions Strategy, Professional: Dawn Gerrain

Director of Content & Business Development, Milady: Sandra Bruce

Senior Acquisitions Editor: Martine Edwards

Senior Product Manager: Jessica Mahoney

Editorial Assistant: Sarah Prediletto

Director, Marketing & Training: Gerard McAvey

Marketing Manager: Matthew McGuire

Senior Production Director: Wendy Troeger

Production Manager: Sherondra Thedford

Senior Content Project Manager: Stacey Lamodi

Senior Art Director: Benj Gleeksman

Cover Images (left to right): © Matka Wariatka/Shutterstock; © Image Source/Corbis; © Yuri Arcurs/Shutterstock

For product information and technology assistance, contact us at
Cengage Learning Customer & Sales Support, 1-800-354-9706
For permission to use material from this text or product,
submit all requests online at **www.cengage.com/permissions.**
Further permissions questions can be e-mailed to
permissionrequest@cengage.com

Library of Congress Control Number: 2012941339

ISBN-13: 978-1-133-60095-4

ISBN-10: 1-133-60095-6

Milady
5 Maxwell Drive
Clifton Park, NY 12065-2919
USA

Cengage Learning is a leading provider of customized learning solutions with office locations around the globe, including Singapore, the United Kingdom, Australia, Mexico, Brazil, and Japan. Locate your local office at:
international.cengage.com/region

Cengage Learning products are represented in Canada by Nelson Education, Ltd.

For your lifelong learning solutions, visit **milady.cengage.com**

Purchase any of our products at your local college store or at our preferred online store **www.cengagebrain.com**

Visit our corporate website at **cengage.com**.

Notice to the Reader

Publisher does not warrant or guarantee any of the products described herein or perform any independent analysis in connection with any of the product information contained herein. Publisher does not assume, and expressly disclaims, any obligation to obtain and include information other than that provided to it by the manufacturer. The reader is expressly warned to consider and adopt all safety precautions that might be indicated by the activities described herein and to avoid all potential hazards. By following the instructions contained herein, the reader willingly assumes all risks in connection with such instructions. The publisher makes no representations or warranties of any kind, including but not limited to, the warranties of fitness for particular purpose or merchantability, nor are any such representations implied with respect to the material set forth herein, and the publisher takes no responsibility with respect to such material. The publisher shall not be liable for any special, consequential, or exemplary damages resulting, in whole or part, from the readers' use of, or reliance upon, this material.

Printed in the United States of America
1 2 3 4 5 6 7 16 15 14 13 12

Table of Contents

Preface

Congratulations for purchasing the *The Visual Guide to Swedish Massage*. This step-by-step manual is a companion text to the *Theory and Practice of Therapeutic Massage*, 5th/6th Edition; however, it may be used as a stand-alone text for those just learning Swedish massage.

The Visual Guide to Swedish Massage is divided into three parts. Part 1 reviews the essential elements of a Swedish massage, including a description of the elementary strokes, how they are applied, draping and the preliminary considerations of preparing the facility, and greeting the client and getting the client comfortably on the table. Part 2 is a step-by-step description of a very basic Swedish massage. This may be a practitioner's first massage and it introduces the practitioner to a simple routine that they can build on in future sessions. Part 3 is a second, more involved Swedish massage routine that adds skills to those learned in the first massage.

Each massage is broken down into areas of the body with descriptions for each step. Each step is illustrated with full-color photographs.

PERFORMANCE RUBRICS

In Parts 2 and 3, rubrics are included, following massage descriptions and illustrations of each body part as a way to note and comment on your performance of each of the key steps. Rubrics are used in education for interpreting and organizing data gathered from observations of student performance. They are scoring documents used to differentiate between levels of development in a specific skill performance or behavior. Students can use rubrics to evaluate themselves or other students to assess where they perform well and where they need more practice. Instructors can use rubrics with students in order to evaluate their progress or possibly adjust curriculum to better serve the students.

ACKNOWLEDGEMENTS

Thank you to each of the following individuals for providing reviewer feedback and contributing their industry knowledge to help us deliver quality content to students, instructors, and professionals.

Stephen Barlow: Colon Hydrotherapist at Every Body Cleansing Studio, Santa Rosa, CA

Felicia Brown: LMBT, Business and Marketing Coach at Spalutions/ Every Touch Marketing, Greensboro, NC

Christi Cano: President of Innovative Spa Products, Las Vegas, NV

Dale Healy: Dean for the School of Massage Therapy at Northwestern Health Sciences University, Bloomington, MN

Kathleen Hunt: Director of Massage Training at Elizabeth Grady School of Esthetics and Massage Therapy, Methuen, MA

Joanne Myers: Cosmetology Instructor, Lancaster, PA

Dale Perry: Licensed Massage Therapist and faculty at CNW School of Massage Therapy, Albany, NY

Kevin Pierce: National Director of Massage Therapy at Anthem Education Group, Orlando, FL

Deborah A. Taylor: Licensed Massage Therapist at East West College of Healing Arts, Portland, OR

Getting Started

The Visual Guide to Swedish Massage will describe and demonstrate how to perform a basic Swedish massage. Before a massage can be performed, there are several considerations to take into account such as the strokes that will be used, the various ways that those strokes are applied, proper draping techniques to assure the clients warmth and modesty, and various pre-service considerations. Part 1 will discuss these topics. Parts 2 and 3 will lead you through two basic massage routines.

Classification of the Basic Swedish Massage Strokes

Massage movements are to therapeutic massage what words are to language or notes to music. To practice massage, an understanding of the movements is imperative. As a massage therapist, the more mastery you have of the movements, the better you can create a work of art each time that you choose and combine movements according to each client's needs. There are any number of massage manipulations and possible combinations of strokes, so that a massage can be tailored to the specific needs of each client. Regardless of whether a massage routine is standard or specialized for the specific needs of the client, there is much more to applying strokes than the movement of the hands. The continuous interaction of the client and therapist, the purpose for the session, and the intent with which each massage stroke is delivered affect the delivery and outcome of the massage.

The following movements are the fundamental massage strokes used in the routine described in the basic *The Visual Guide to Swedish Massage*. A more comprehensive description of massage strokes is found in the *Theory and Practice of Therapeutic Massage*. The massage practitioner must understand the indications for, and effects of, each massage stroke. The intention with which a massage is given or a technique is applied greatly influences its effect. Each manipulation is applied in a specific way for a particular purpose. The practice of massage becomes scientific only when the practitioner recognizes the purpose and effects of each movement and adapts the treatment to the client's condition for the desired results.

EFFLEURAGE OR GLIDING

Effleurage, or **gliding**, is the practice of sliding the hand or forearm over a portion of the client's body, with varying amounts of pressure or contact according to the desired results. Effleurage is perhaps the most frequently used movement in Swedish or Western massage. There are two varieties of effleurage: superficial and deep.

Superficial gliding

Superficial gliding strokes are generally applied prior to any other movement. The practitioner's hand is flexible yet firm and controlled so that as it slides smoothly over the body, it conforms to the body contours so that there is equal pressure applied to the body from every part of the hand. Light strokes are used to distribute any lubricant that is used and to prepare the area for other techniques. Superficial gliding strokes accustom the client to the practitioner's contact and allow the practitioner to assess the body area being massaged. As the practitioner's hands glide over the tissues, they sense variations that indicate where specific techniques should be applied (**Figure 1-1**). Effleurage is

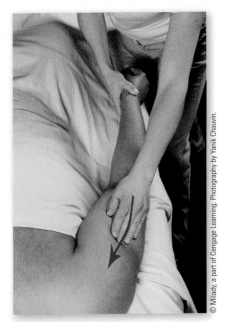

© Milady, a part of Cengage Learning. Photography by Yanik Chauvin.

▲ **FIGURE 1–1**
Superficial effleurage on the arm is in the direction of venous and lymph flow.

interspersed with other techniques to clear the area and soothe the intensity of some deeper movements. In Swedish or Western massage, effleurage is generally the first and the last technique used on an area of the body. Slow, gentle, and rhythmic movements produce soothing effects. Rhythmic strokes should be applied in the direction of the venous and lymphatic flow (**Figure 1-2**).

On the extremities, the gliding stroke can be continuous, with slightly more pressure toward the heart and very light pressure on the return stroke.

Deep gliding

The term **deep gliding** indicates that the movement uses enough pressure to have a mechanical effect. The depth of the gliding movement depends on three factors: the pressure exerted, the part of the hand or arm used, and the intention with which the movement is applied. Deep gliding can be applied with the hand, thumb, braced fingers, knuckles, or forearm, depending on the area of the body or tissues involved (**Figures 1-3 to 1-5**). Deep gliding strokes do not involve the use of excessive force, however. The pressure should never be forceful enough to cause bruising or injury to the tissues. Deep gliding strokes are especially valuable when applied to the muscles and are most effective when the part undergoing treatment is in a relaxed state. The slightest pressure of the surface is then transmitted to the deeper structures. The movement is usually toward the heart or in the direction of venous and lymph flow, with the return stroke being much lighter and away from the center of the body.

When using deep gliding strokes, the practitioner must use good body mechanics to prevent strain and overuse syndrome injuries. The practitioner's movement should come from the body core. The practitioner's shoulders remain down and relaxed, with the wrists, fingers, or thumbs in proper alignment. Hyperextension of any joint must be avoided. When applying long, gliding strokes, the practitioner should shift weight from the back foot to the front foot or take small steps to distribute body weight and maintain consistent pressure throughout the length of the stroke.

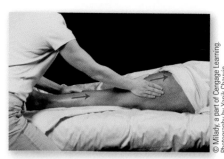

▲ FIGURE 1-2
Superficial effleurage on the leg can cover the length of the limb.

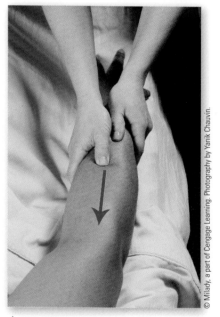

▲ FIGURE 1-3
Deep gliding using the thumb.

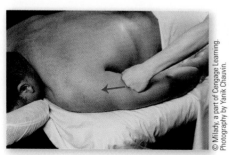

▲ FIGURE 1-4
Deep gliding using a loose fist.

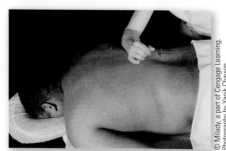

▲ FIGURE 1-5
Deep gliding using the forearm.

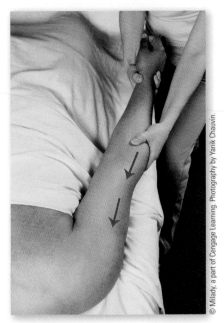

▲ FIGURE 1–6
A V-stroke can be used for superficial or deep gliding.

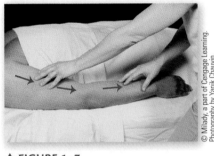

▲ FIGURE 1–7
Feather strokes.

V-stroke

The V-stroke is a gliding stroke where the practitioner's hand is held in such a way that the thumb is abducted to form a "V" with the first finger (**Figure 1-6**). The hand glides along the target tissue so the thumb and first finger encircle the target tissue as the stroke glides in the direction of lymph and venous flow. The V-stroke can be used for superficial or deep gliding strokes.

Feather strokes

Feather strokes use very light pressure of the fingertips or hands, with long, flowing strokes (**Figure 1-7**).

The application of feather strokes, sometimes called *nerve strokes*, is usually done from the center outward and is used as a final stroke to individual areas of the body. Two or three such strokes have a slightly stimulating effect on the nerves, whereas many repetitions have a more sedating response.

PETRISSAGE OR KNEADING

Kneading lifts, squeezes, and presses the tissues. In Swedish massage, kneading or **petrissage** is used on all fleshy areas of the body. Like deep gliding, kneading enhances the fluid movement in the deeper tissues and can help break up superficial adhesions. In this movement, the skin and muscular tissues are raised from their ordinary position and then squeezed, rolled, or kneaded with a firm pressure, usually in a circular direction (**Figure 1-8**).

On large areas of the body, both hands work alternately as a unit. The tissue is lifted with the palmar surface of the fingers of one hand into the palm of the other hand. Then the process is reversed so that the fingers of the other hand lift the tissue into the palm and base of the opposite hand. The hands alternate in a rhythmic circular pattern over the entire body part being massaged.

Over smaller structures, such as the arms or legs, the flesh is grasped between the fingers and heel of the hand or the thumb (**Figure 1-9**). In both cases, the maximum amount of flesh is drawn up into the palm and gently and firmly pressed and squeezed, as if milking the tissues.

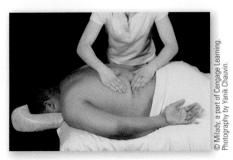

▲ FIGURE 1–8
Petrissage.

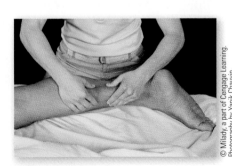

▲ FIGURE 1–9
Kneading the calf muscles.

On an area such as the arm, one hand can be used to apply the movement while the other hand stabilizes the arm, or both hands can alternate, grasping the tissue on each side of the arm (**Figure 1-10**).

On even smaller structures, such as the fingers or toes, the flesh is kneaded between the practitioner's thumb and fingers (**Figure 1-11**).

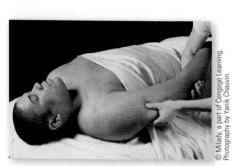

▲ FIGURE 1–10
Kneading the triceps and biceps.

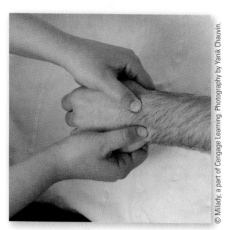

▲ FIGURE 1–11
Petrissage of the wrist and hand.

Fulling

Fulling is a kneading technique in which the practitioner attempts to grasp the tissue and gently lift and spread it out, as if to make more space between the layers of tissue or muscle fibers (**Figure 1-12**). Fulling is applied to the muscular areas of the arm or leg. Often done with both hands simultaneously, the fleshy body part is gathered up between two hands, then raised and separated by the thenar eminence (fleshy part of the palm of the hand near the thumb) and thumbs as the part is gently stretched across the fibers of the tissue.

FRICTION

Friction refers to several massage strokes designed to manipulate soft tissue in such a way that one layer of tissue is moved over or against another. *Friction movements* involve moving more superficial layers of flesh against the deeper tissues. This requires pressure on the skin while it is being moved over its underlying structures. The skin and the practitioner's hand move as a unit against the deeper tissue. Friction is performed in such a way that it also increases heat. The added heat and energy affect the connective tissue surrounding the muscles, making them more pliable so that they function more efficiently.

Circular friction

In **circular friction**, the pads of the fingers or the thumb contact the skin to move it in a circular pattern over the deeper tissues (**Figure 1-13**). Circular friction, which is intended to produce heat and stretch and soften the fascia, is a general stroke used to warm the area in preparation

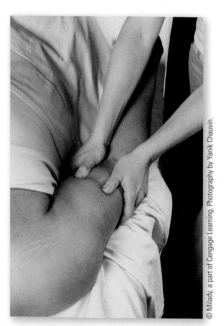

▲ FIGURE 1–12
Fulling movement.

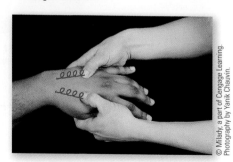

▲ FIGURE 1–13
Circular friction using the thumbs on the hand.

for more specific or deeper work. When performing circular friction, the fingers or hand do not slide over the skin in a circular manner. The intent is to move the superficial layer of tissue over a deeper layer, resulting in a gentle stretching and warming of the area (**Figure 1-14**).

Circular friction is also valuable for palpating an area when assessing the condition of the underlying tissues. When working deeply on an area, circular friction and superficial gliding strokes are useful to soothe and calm the client before, after, and interspersed with deep techniques (**Figure 1-15**).

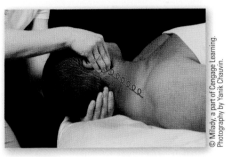

▲ FIGURE 1–14
Circular friction using the fingers on the back of the neck.

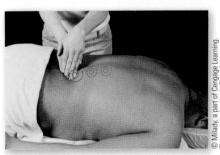

▲ FIGURE 1–15
Circular friction using braced fingers on the thicker tissues on the back.

Wringing

Wringing is a back-and-forth movement in which both of the practitioner's hands are placed a short distance apart on either side of the limb. The movement resembles that of wringing out a washcloth. The hands work in opposing directions, stretching and twisting the flesh against the bones in opposite directions (**Figure 1-16**). The practitioner's whole body is engaged in the movement, and the hands make firm contact in both directions. Pressure is not excessive enough to cause pinching or burning (irritation) of the skin, however. Wringing gently stretches and warms the connective fascia (**Figure 1-17**).

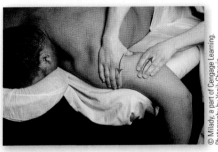

▲ FIGURE 1–16
Wringing the muscles of the arm.

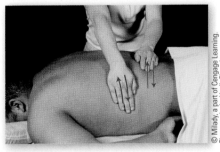

▲ FIGURE 1–17
Wringing the muscles of the lower back.

Rolling

Rolling is a rapid back-and-forth movement with the hands, in which the flesh is shaken and rolled around the *axis*, or the imaginary centerline, of the body part (**Figures 1-18 and 1-19**). The intention of rolling is to warm and relax the tissue. Rolling encourages deep muscle relaxation.

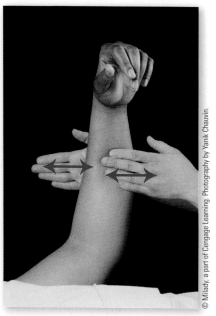

▲ FIGURE 1–18
Rolling the muscles of the arm.

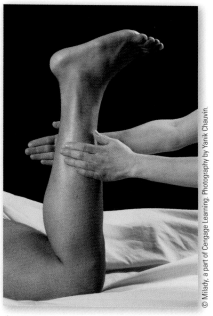

▲ FIGURE 1–19
Rolling the muscles of the lower leg.

PASSIVE JOINT MOVEMENTS

Joint movement is the passive or active movement of the joints or articulations of the client. A great variety of joint movements can be used to move any joint in the body, including joints of the toes, knees, hips, arms, and vertebrae.

Passive joint movements (PJM) are done while the client remains quietly relaxed and allow the practitioner to stretch and move the part of the body to be exercised **(Figure 1-20)**. PJM can be used as an assessment tool to determine normal movement (full range of motion without restriction or pain). These movements gently stretch the fibrous connective tissue and move the joint through its range of motion. PJMs are used therapeutically to improve joint mobility and range of motion, always working within the client's comfort level.

When performing PJMs, hold and support the limb so that the movement is directed toward the target joint **(Figure 1-21)**. Move the limb in a normal movement pattern for that joint. Move the limb to the full extent of possible movement within the client's comfort level. If the movement is for assessment purposes, move only to the point of resistance and note the extent and quality of the movement. If the movement is therapeutic, challenge the range of movement by slightly extending or pushing into the end of the movement.

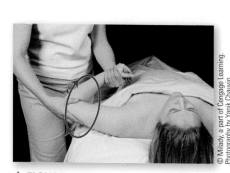

▲ FIGURE 1–20
Circumducting the shoulder by moving the elbow in large circles.

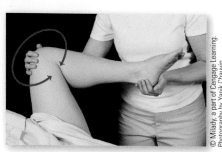

▲ FIGURE 1–21
Passive joint movements of the leg.

PERCUSSION

Percussion is a rapid striking motion of the practitioner's hands against the surface of the client's body, using varying amounts of force and hand positions.

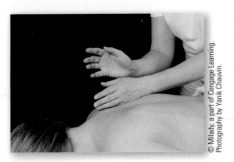

▲ FIGURE 1–22
Hacking movements on the back.

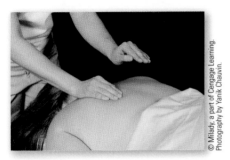

▲ FIGURE 1–23
Cupping movements on the back.

Hacking

Hacking encourages relaxation and local circulation. Some theories claim that hacking stimulates the nerve responses in muscles and helps to firm the muscles. Hacking is a rapid striking movement that can be done with one or both hands (**Figure 1-22**). When both hands are used, the hands can strike alternately or together. A quick glancing strike is made with the little finger and the ulnar side of the hand. The wrist and fingers remain loose and relaxed, and the fingers are slightly spread apart. As the side of the hand strikes the body, the fingers come together, causing a slight vibrating effect.

Cupping

Cupping is a technique often employed by respiratory therapists to help break up lung congestion and is usually done over the rib cage. To perform cupping, form a cup of the hands by keeping the fingers together and slightly flexed with the thumb held close to the side of the palm (**Figure 1-23**). On each percussion the perimeter of the hand contacts the skin, producing a hollow popping sound.

Slapping

Slapping is applied with the palmar surface of the fingers and palm and produces a crisp "smacking" sound when done correctly (**Figure 1-24**). Slapping is very stimulating and must be used sparingly. Slapping encourages local peripheral circulation and gives a "glow" to the area.

Beating

Beating is the heaviest and deepest form of percussion and is used over the thicker, denser, and fleshier areas of the body (**Figure 1-25**). The hands are held in a loose fist. The therapist makes contact with the ulnar aspect of both hands either together or alternately. The wrists are relaxed so that the contact is the result of a rebounding, whiplike action of the hand and wrist. The force is never heavy or hard.

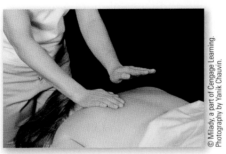

▲ FIGURE 1–24
Slapping movements on the back.

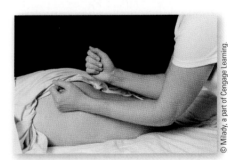

▲ FIGURE 1–25
Beating the thicker gluteal muscles.

Classification of Basic Massage Strokes

Rubrics are used in education for organizing and interpreting data gathered from observations of student performance. It is a clearly developed scoring document used to differentiate between levels of development in a specific skill performance or behavior. Rubrics are provided in this supplement for use as either a self-assessment tool to aid the student in behavior development or as an educator assessment tool to determine competence. Space is provided to record steps needed for further growth and improvement.

Performance is evaluated according to the following scale:

1 **Development Opportunity**: There is little or no evidence of competency; Assistance is needed; Performance includes multiple errors.

2 **Fundamental**: There is beginning evidence of competency; Task is completed alone; Performance includes few errors.

3 **Competent**: There is detailed and consistent evidence of competency; Task is completed alone; Performance includes rare errors.

4 **Strength**: There is detailed evidence of highly creative, inventive, mature presence of competency.

Space is provided for comments to assist you in improving your performance and achieving a higher rating.

PERFORMANCE ASSESSED	1	2	3	4	IMPROVEMENT PLAN
Procedure					
1. Demonstrated superficial gliding strokes on two areas of the body.					
2. Demonstrated deep gliding strokes using the thumb.					
3. Demonstrated deep gliding strokes using a loose fist.					
4. Demonstrated deep gliding strokes using the forearm.					
5. Demonstrated a V-stroke on the arm or leg.					
6. Demonstrated a feather stroke on the arm or leg.					
7. Demonstrated petrissage on the back.					
8. Demonstrated petrissage on a leg.					
9. Demonstrated petrissage on an arm.					
10. Demonstrated petrissage on the hand.					
11. Demonstrated fulling on the back of the leg.					
12. Demonstrated circular friction on the hand.					
13. Demonstrated circular friction on the neck.					
14. Demonstrated circular friction on the back.					
15. Demonstrated wringing on the back.					
16. Demonstrated wringing on the arm or leg.					
17. Demonstrated rolling on the arm.					
18. Demonstrated rolling on the leg.					

PERFORMANCE ASSESSED	1	2	3	4	IMPROVEMENT PLAN
19. Demonstrated passive joint movements on the arm.					
20. Demonstrated passive joint movements on the leg.					
21. Demonstrated hacking on the back.					
22. Demonstrated cupping over the area of the lungs.					
23. Demonstrated slapping on the back.					
24. Demonstrated beating over the gluteal muscles.					

Notes

Application of Massage Movements

The manner in which the basic massage strokes are applied determines the effect they have on the person. Intention, direction, speed, length, duration, and pressure of the stroke each play a part in the effect it has on the individual. The sequence of the massage pertains to the organization of the overall treatment as well as how each body part is addressed. The practitioner controls these various qualities according to the condition and wishes of the client and the purpose of the massage.

INTENTION

Intention is a mental process of consciously holding a desired goal or outcome in mind when engaging in or performing an activity. When performing a massage, the intention is influenced by the wishes and needs of the client as well as the desired outcome of each movement and the treatment as a whole (**Figure 2-1**). An infant massage will have a very different intention than a sports massage (**Figure 2-2**). The intention of the massages described in this text is relaxation so most of the strokes therefore will be to relax the tissues. That intention will influence how the following attributes will be applied.

DIRECTION

The direction of a stroke helps determine its influence on the underlying tissues. Strokes toward the heart encourage venous blood and lymph circulation, reduce edema, and tend to be relaxing and soothing (**Figure 2-3**). Strokes away from the heart or into the tissues tend to be more stimulating and energizing (**Figure 2-4**).

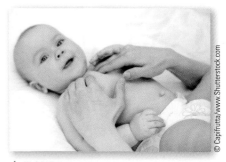
▲ FIGURE 2–1
The intention of an infant massage is to sooth and connect.

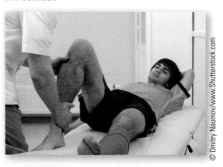
▲ FIGURE 2–2
The intention of a sports massage may be to stimulate and stretch or relax depending on the situation.

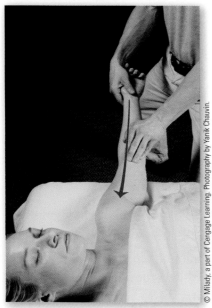
▲ FIGURE 2–3
Long strokes toward the heart tend to be relaxing and soothing.

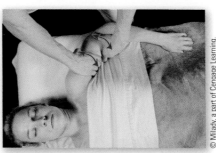
▲ FIGURE 2–4
Short strokes across the muscle fiber direction tend to strech the tissue and soften adhesions.

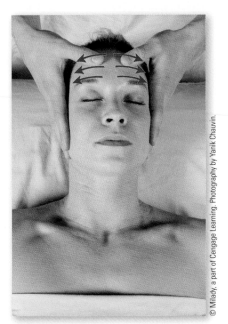
▲ FIGURE 2–5
Gliding strokes on the face are very short.

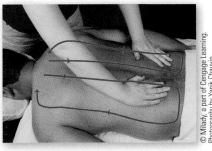
▲ FIGURE 2–6
Gliding strokes on the back or limbs can be very long or quite short depending on the intention.

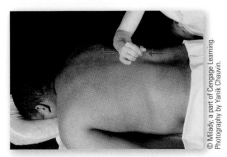
▲ FIGURE 2–7
Deeper pressure can be applied with the forearm, elbow, soft fist, or braced thumb.

Strokes across the fiber orientation of the tissues tend to stretch the tissue and soften adhesions.

SPEED

The speed with which a particular stroke is delivered is partially determined by the intention of the massage and in particular the intention of the individual stroke. Quicker strokes will be more invigorating and stimulating. Slower, more rhythmic strokes tend to be more relaxing. Most of the techniques in this text are intended to be relaxing therefore tend to be relatively slow and rhythmical.

LENGTH

The length or excursion is how far the stroke travels over the body. This particularly applies to gliding or effleurage. The stroke can be as short as an inch (2.54 cm) or two inches (5.08 cm) and concentrate on a part of the hand, neck, or face (**Figure 2-5**). Or the stroke can glide over the entire length of an arm, leg, or the back (**Figure 2-6**). On the arm or leg for instance, the first strokes can cover the entire length of the limb, followed by several shorter gliding strokes concentrated on particular segments of the limb.

DURATION

Duration refers to how long or the number of times a stroke is done on a particular area. Duration could also refer to the amount of time using a variety of strokes on a particular area of the body. Spending too much time on an area might be fatiguing or result in soreness. Of course, the combination of all of the strokes given during a session determines the duration of the entire massage. The time spent on each area should be monitored so there is adequate time to address all the areas of the body that are intended within a suitable time frame for the massage. The duration of a full body massage should be in the neighborhood of an hour.

DEPTH/PRESSURE

The amount of force the practitioner applies against the client's body with their hands, thumbs, fingers, or elbows determines the pressure of the stroke. Pressure is controlled by the practitioner according to the intention of and the type of stroke used. The way pressure is applied affects its intensity:

- When applied with the broad surface of the hand or forearm, it is more defused and tends to be soothing and relaxing (**Figure 2-7**).

- When applied with the thumbs, knuckles, or point of the elbow, the pressure is more concentrated, deep, and intense.

Caution must be used to assure the amount of pressure applied does not cause too much pain or discomfort. Many times clients seek massage services because they are experiencing pain. As the massage proceeds over the areas of concern, the client may experience a certain amount of discomfort that "hurts good" as the practitioner works out the congestion and tension in the tissues. This level of discomfort is expected. However, the practitioner must use good judgment and open communication with the client to not cross the client's "pain threshold." If the pain threshold is crossed, the client will pull back, tighten up, and possibly lose trust in the practitioner and the massage process. This is counterproductive to the whole massage process. It is important for the practitioner to observe the client's facial expressions or body reactions and to ask the client how the pressure is and make any necessary adjustments.

The **depth** of a massage stroke refers to how deep into the tissues the effects of a particular stroke reaches. The depth is determined by a number of factors, among them, the intention of the movement, the type of movement, and the condition and quality of the tissues to which the movement is being directed.

As mentioned earlier, the intention of a movement is the initial determinant of what movement is chosen for what purpose. The intention also creates a mental energy as to the intent of the outcome of a particular treatment. When the intention is to affect the more superficial or the deeper tissues, the energy of the movement is directed toward those tissues.

The selection of a massage movement, the amount of pressure used in the application of that movement, and the direction of the movement each play a part in the depth of the movement.

The quality and condition of the target tissues help determine the depth of any particular movement. If, for instance, the area being massaged is contracted and tense, the depth of the massage will be sustained in those tissues. If, however, the underlying tissues are more relaxed and supple, the depth of the movement can move down through those tissues. More pressure does not necessarily result in deeper massage. The practitioner must take into account the condition of the tissues and then apply the selected movement with the appropriate pressure to obtain the optimal depth and desired outcome according to the goals of the treatment (**Figure 2-8**).

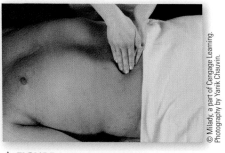

▲ FIGURE 2–8
The depth of a massage technique depends as much on the condition of the underlying target tissue as on the pressure used.

© Milady, a part of Cengage Learning. Photography by Yanik Chauvin.

SEQUENCE

Sequence refers to the pattern or design of a massage. Developing a good sequence is especially important because it coordinates and organizes the massage so that there is smooth progression from one stroke to the next and from one body part to the next. Sequence provides a framework for a well-thought-out, logical progression and at the same time allows for flexibility and creativity. When doing a full-body massage, following a sequence ensures that each and every area of the body is massaged in a logical order.

There are numerous possibilities when formulating a full-body massage sequence, depending on the style of the practitioner, the preferences and needs of the client, and the intentions of the session, among many other considerations. The sequence can begin with the client lying face up, face down, or on their side. The massage can begin at the head, at the feet, or somewhere in between. Generally, a Western- or Swedish-style massage is designed so that the client only has to change positions once or maybe twice. A relaxing, wellness massage sequence is designed so that each body area is thoroughly massaged in a logical order so that the entire body is included and the client feels balanced, complete, and relaxed. Some therapeutic applications require the therapist to focus on specific areas of the client's body or to return to an area several times during a session but not even approach other areas of the body. In so doing, the therapist is following a sequence to address the specific needs of the client efficiently. Even in a relaxing full-body massage, the sequence is a guideline that is always flexible enough for the individual needs of the client to be addressed.

Following a massage sequence on a particular body area provides a structure that you, the practitioner, can use to ensure a balanced and complete therapeutic application to that area. In the application of a massage, sequences are built within sequences, and each body part is provided an equal experience. Even during the massage of a body part, there are conditions in which adapting a certain sequence proves both valuable and therapeutic.

There is a general massage rule to keep in mind. When doing massage, performing a stroke, or working on an area:

Work from general to specific, then back to general, and from superficial to deep and back to superficial.

In working from general to specific, the entire area is relaxed and local circulation is increased so that more specific massage can relieve congestion and spasm. Ischemic conditions also have a better chance of being relieved. Following specific massage techniques with more generalized massage tends to normalize the area.

Likewise, starting with more superficial effleurage or gliding strokes relaxes the area and encourages the client's confidence to let you work more deeply into the tissues. Following deeper massage techniques, soothing superficial gliding strokes dissipate the tension released from the target tissues and enhance a sense of relaxation.

The sequence of the overall massage is designed in a logical progression that leaves the client with a feeling of completeness. Although a sequence might vary according to the situation, a pattern should be used that ensures that every part of the body is massaged properly and thoroughly.

Massage movements for adjacent areas as well as bilateral body parts should follow in sequence. For example, when beginning with the hand, the massage should progress to the arm and then to the shoulder.

GENERAL MASSAGE RULE

When working on an area or performing a stroke, work from general to specific then back to general,

AND

work from superficial to deep then back to superficial

Then massage the other hand, arm, and shoulder, both shoulders, the neck, and the head. Finally, massage the chest, abdomen, one leg and foot, and then the other leg and foot. This completes the massage for the front of the body.

Developing a sequence also ensures a thorough massage that is balanced between one body part and another. The following is an example of an effective sequence to be used on each body area when giving a relaxing wellness massage.

1. Make contact with and undrape the body part to be massaged.

2. Apply massage lubricant with light effleurage.

3. Apply effleurage to accustom the body to your touch. Effleurage also enhances local circulation.

4. Apply petrissage, kneading the tissues to warm them. This also enables you to become aware of any areas of tension or congestion in the muscles.

5. Apply effleurage to flush the area.

6. Apply friction with any of the recommended friction techniques.

7. Apply deep gliding strokes to areas that seem especially tight or congested.

8. Apply effleurage to the entire area again, flushing the area while linking and integrating the segmented parts back into the whole.

9. Do joint movements to restore mobility by reinforcing the possibility of movement. At the same time, joint movements stretch the muscles and connective tissues and lubricate the joints.

10. Apply effleurage to flush out the area and to give a feeling of length to the body part.

11. Apply feather strokes. This stimulates the peripheral nervous system, smoothes the energy field, and says good-bye to that part of the body.

12. Re-drape the part of the body that has been massaged, undrape the next part, and continue until the client has been given a thorough massage.

Draping Procedures

IMPLEMENTS AND MATERIALS FOR DRAPING

You will need all of the following implements, materials, and supplies:

- Massage table (with face rest)
- Cot-size fitted sheets or twin-sized flat sheets for a table covering.
- One-half of full double sheets, cut and hemmed or twin-sized flat sheets to use as a table covering or a cover sheet.
- Disposable sheets to use as table coverings when laundry is a problem

- Variety of bolsters and pillows
- Pillowcases for covering pillows and bolsters
- Washcloths, pillow covers, or specifically manufactured protectors to cover face cradles
- Flannel sheets or light cotton blanket to use when extra warmth is needed

Overview

The process of using linens to keep a client covered while performing a massage is called **draping**. By using proper draping (uncovering only the portion of the body that is being massaged) and by always concealing the client's private parts, the practitioner maintains a professional and ethical practice while preventing embarrassment to either the practitioner or the client.

Several methods of draping are easy and effective. In *The Visual Guide to Swedish Massage*, we will use the **top cover method** of draping. The top cover method uses a table covering along with a top covering that is large enough to cover the entire body. A large bath sheet towel, one-half of a double sheet, or a twin-sized sheet will serve this purpose well. The minimum size for the top cover is 72 inches (182.88 cm) long and 36 inches (91.44 cm) wide. The cover sheet may also serve as the wrap the client uses to get from the dressing area to the table.

The use of this type of draping ensures warmth and modesty while allowing easy access to each body part. Remember that any materials coming in contact with the client's skin must be freshly laundered. Clean linens must be used for each client.

Some clients cannot comfortably lie on the back or face down without support. For these clients, it is helpful to have foam cushions and bolsters in various shapes and sizes **(Figure 3-1)**. These are made of fairly high-density foam and are covered with vinyl for easy cleaning. Pillows or folded towels can also be used to position the client for comfort.

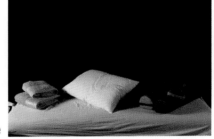

▲ FIGURE 3−1
A variety of bolsters and pillows.

Bolsters as wide as the table and 4 (10.16 cm to 20.32 cm) to 8 inches in diameter can be used under the client's knees when the client is lying on their back to place the lower spine in a more relaxed position **(Figure 3-2)**.

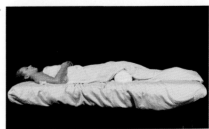

▲ FIGURE 3−2
A bolster behind the knee reduces tension in the back of the legs and the low back.

A bolster placed under the ankles when the client is lying face down prevents hyperextension of the knees and ankles and relieves tension in the lower back (**Figure 3-3**).

Bolsters should be covered with a pillowcase or placed under the sheets or draping material so that they do not come in direct contact with the client's skin. Firm bed pillows can also be used.

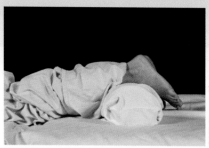

▲ FIGURE 3–3
A bolster under the ankles relieves tension in the lower back.

When it is time to begin, the practitioner accompanies the client into the massage studio (or area) and prepares the massage table with a table covering and a top sheet or large towel. The client is instructed to remove her clothing, lay on the table in the chosen position, and cover herself with the appropriate drape. The practitioner then leaves the room. The client disrobes, climbs on the table, and covers herself. It is important to give concise, yet simple, instructions so that the client is in the correct position and properly covered when the practitioner re-enters the massage room.

When the massage is complete, the practitioner may instruct the client to take a few minutes to relax and then carefully get up and get dressed. The practitioner then exits the room and leaves the client on her own to get off the massage table and to get dressed.

If there is any concern that the client may need some assistance getting up at the end of the session, the practitioner should remain in the massage room to assist the client to a sitting position and then off the table before leaving the room and allowing the client privacy to dress. Use proper draping techniques to ensure that the client remains modestly covered as she sits up and gets off the table.

Draping Procedures continued

Top Cover Method

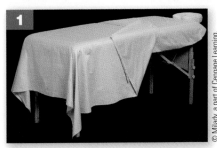

1 Prepare the massage table by completely covering the table with a sheet. Arrange a second sheet as a top cover so it covers the lower three-quarters of the table and is turned down.

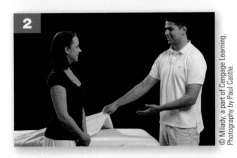

2 Instruct the client to disrobe and lie face-up on the table and cover herself with the top sheet. Then leave the room as the client gets undressed and situated on the table.

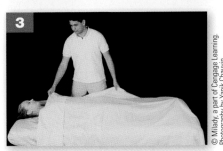

3 When the client is on the table, return to the room and situate the top cover lengthwise to cover all except her head.

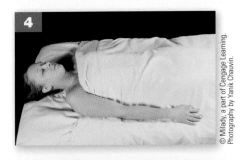

4 Undrape an arm by lifting the side of the wrap enough to grasp the client's hand, pull the hand and arm from under the cover, and then place it on top of the drape. Replace the arm and hand under the drape when finished massaging them.

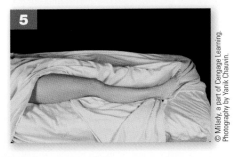

5 To massage a leg, uncover that leg only. Lift the knee enough to reach under and pull the drape under the thigh and toward the buttock with one hand while positioning the cover snugly across the upper thigh with your other hand.

6 To massage the chest and abdomen of a man, neatly fold the top cover to the level of the hips. A bolster may be placed under the knees to further relax the abdomen.

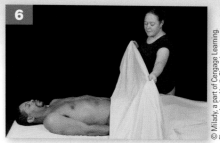

Breast Draping

7 To work on the abdomen of a woman, breast draping is needed. Fold another towel or pillowcase to make a covering for the breasts and place it over the top cover.

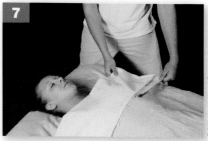

8 Peel the top cover down while holding the folded towel or pillowcase in place over the breasts.

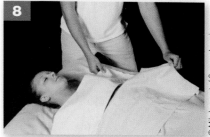

9 Place the client's arm down. Tuck the other side of the towel or pillowcase covering the breasts under the arm or the scapula in the same manner. This draping method allows you to work on the abdomen, chest, and sides of the body without exposing the breasts.

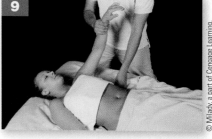

10 Raise the client's arm and tuck the towel or pillowcase used for the breast cover neatly under the arm or the scapula to hold the ends of the towel securely in place.

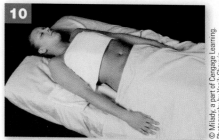

Draping Procedures continued

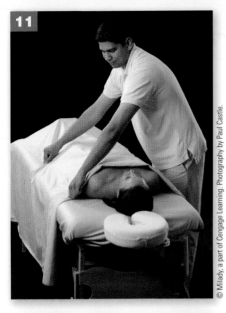

11 When it is time to roll over, the drape is repositioned and held in place by the therapist leaning on the table and grasping the top cover at the level of the client's shoulders and hips.

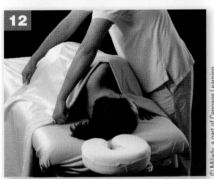

12 When rolling from supine to prone, the client is instructed to roll first to face the therapist and then onto her stomach.

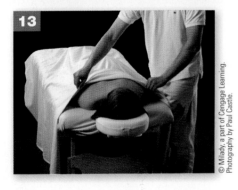

13 Instruct the client to slide up on the table to comfortably position their face in the face cradle and adjust the draping to cover the body from the neck down.

14 Undrape one leg, beginning at the foot and exposing the leg. Tuck the drape under the opposite thigh and secure the drape as you uncover the gluteal area up to the ilium. Secure the drape, being careful not to expose the gluteal cleft.

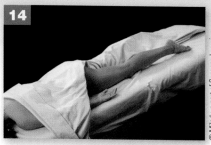

© Milady, a part of Cengage Learning. Photography by Paul Castle.

15 To massage the back, neatly fold the top cover down to a level no more than two inches below the beginning of the gluteal cleft.

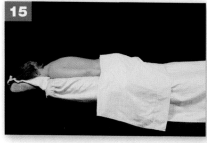

© Milady, a part of Cengage Learning. Photography by Yanik Chauvin.

16 When the massage is complete re-drape the back and instruct the client to rest for a moment then carefully get off of the table and dressed. If there is any concern the client may need assistance getting off the table, follow the next steps.

Assisting the Client Off the Table

17 To assist the client into a sitting position and off of the table, adjust the top cover so that it covers the client from her shoulders down to at least mid-thigh.

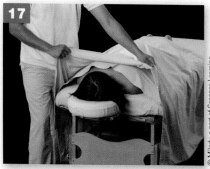

© Milady, a part of Cengage Learning. Photography by Paul Castle.

18 Instruct the client to turn onto her side and bend her knees. Allow the top cover to wrap around the client as she turns.

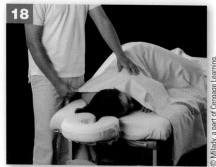

© Milady, a part of Cengage Learning. Photography by Paul Castle.

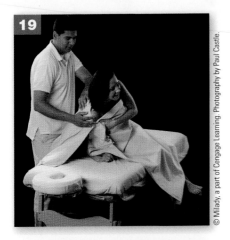

© Milady, a part of Cengage Learning. Photography by Paul Castle.

19 From this side-lying position, instruct the client to sit up while securing the top sheet. Assist the client into a sitting position by lifting her shoulder. Secure the top sheet for use as a wrap.

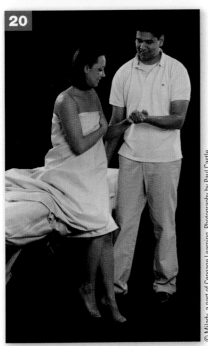

© Milady, a part of Cengage Learning. Photography by Paul Castle.

20 After a moment, when the client has regained alertness, assist her off the table into a standing position by keeping one hand on the client and the other on the table to steady both. A step stool may be used if the table is too tall for the client to safely step on or off. Instruct the client to get dressed as you leave the room.

Draping Procedures

Rubrics are used in education for organizing and interpreting data gathered from observations of student performance. It is a clearly developed scoring document used to differentiate between levels of development in a specific skill performance or behavior. Rubrics are provided in this supplement for use as either a self-assessment tool to aid the student in behavior development or as an educator assessment tool to determine competence. Space is provided to record steps needed for further growth and improvement.

Performance is evaluated according to the following scale:

1 **Development Opportunity**: There is little or no evidence of competency; Assistance is needed; Performance includes multiple errors.

2 **Fundamental**: There is beginning evidence of competency; Task is completed alone; Performance includes few errors.

3 **Competent**: There is detailed and consistent evidence of competency; Task is completed alone; Performance includes rare errors.

4 **Strength**: There is detailed evidence of highly creative, inventive, mature presence of competency. Space is provided for comments to assist you in improving your performance and achieving a higher rating.

PERFORMANCE ASSESSED	1	2	3	4	IMPROVEMENT PLAN
Procedure					
1. Prepared the massage table with a table covering and a top sheet. The top sheet covers the lower ¾ of the table and is turned down.					
2. Instructed the client to disrobe, lay face-up on the table, and cover themselves with the top sheet. Then left the room as the client got dressed and situated on the table.					
3. Returned to the room. Adjusted the top sheet when the client was on the table.					
4a. Undraped one arm by slightly lifting the side of the drape and putting the arm on top of the drape.					
4b. Re-draped the arm.					
5a. Undraped one leg from the hip to the crest of the ilium.					
5b. Tucked the drape in such a way to conceal the genitals.					
5c. Re-draped the leg.					
6. Undraped the chest and abdomen of a male client. OR Applied breast draping on a female client.					
For Breast Draping					
7. Folded another towel or pillowcase to make a covering for the breasts and placed it over the top cover.					

PERFORMANCE ASSESSED	1	2	3	4	IMPROVEMENT PLAN
8. Peeled the top cover down while holding the folded towel or pillowcase in place over the breasts.					
9. Raised the client's arm and tucked the towel or pillowcase used for the breast cover neatly under the scapula to hold the ends of the towel securely in place.					
10. Placed the client's arm down. Tucked the other side of the towel or pillowcase covering the breasts under the other scapula in the same manner.					
11–12. Held the draping and instructed the client to roll from supine to prone.					
13. Instructed the client to slide up on the table to comfortably position their face in the face cradle and adjusted the draping to cover the body from the neck down.					
14a. Undraped one leg, including the gluteal area.					
14b. Re-draped the leg.					
15. Undraped the back.					
16a. Re-draped the back.					
16b. Assisted the client to a sitting position, maintaining proper draping.					
Assisting the Client Off the Table					
17. Adjusted the top cover so that it covers the client from their shoulders down to at least mid-thigh.					
18. Instructed the client to turn onto their side and bend their knees. Allowed the top cover to wrap around the client as they turned.					
19. From the side-lying position, instructed the client and assisted them to sit up while securing the top sheet. Secured the top sheet to be used as a wrap.					
20. When the client regained alertness, assisted them off the table into a standing position by keeping one hand on the client and the other on the table to steady both. A step stool may be used.					

Pre-Service Procedure

IMPLEMENTS AND MATERIALS (USE THIS LIST FOR ALL MASSAGE PROCEDURES)

- Massage table (with head rest)
- Stool or chair
- Variety of lubricants
- Cot-size fitted sheets for a table covering or one-half of full double sheets, cut and hemmed or twin-sized flat sheets to use as a table covering or a cover sheet
- Disposable sheets to use as table coverings when laundry is a problem

- Variety of bolsters and pillows
- Pillowcases for covering pillows and bolsters
- Washcloths, pillow covers, or specifically manufactured protectors to cover face cradles
- Flannel sheets to use when extra warmth is needed

Preparing the Treatment Room

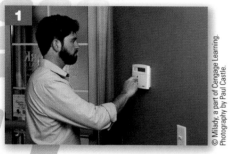

© Milady, a part of Cengage Learning. Photography by Paul Castle.

1 Prepare the facility. Make sure the premises are clean and at a comfortable temperature. The proper temperature for a massage room is between 72° F and 75° F (22.22° C and 23.88° C).

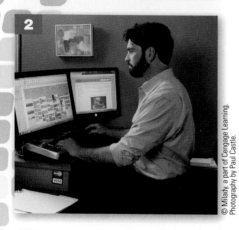

© Milady, a part of Cengage Learning. Photography by Paul Castle.

2 Review your client schedule for the day and decide on which materials and products you are likely to need. Make sure you have enough of all materials and products you will be using that day. This is also a good time to refresh your mind about each client you will be seeing that day and his or her individual concerns.

Pre-Service Procedure continued

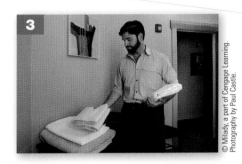

© Milady, a part of Cengage Learning. Photography by Paul Castle.

3 Check your room supply of linens (towels and sheets) and replenish as needed.

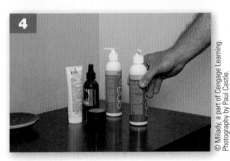

© Milady, a part of Cengage Learning. Photography by Paul Castle.

4 Select the lubricants that will be used. A wide variety of lubricants are available. The practitioner should choose a lubricant that will allow the hands to glide smoothly over the client's skin. Use a container that is easy to access the product without contaminating the contents.

Preparing for the Client

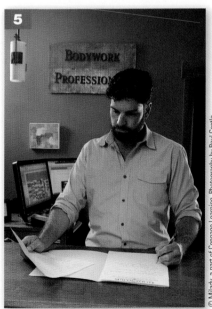

© Milady, a part of Cengage Learning. Photography by Paul Castle.

5 Retrieve the client's file with intake and medical history forms and review it. If the appointment is for a new client, let the front desk receptionist know that the client will need an intake form.

6 Organize yourself by taking care of personal needs before the client arrives—use the restroom, get a drink of water, return a personal call—so that when your client arrives, you can place your full attention on her needs.

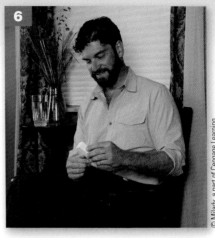

7 Turn off your cell phone, pager, or PDA. Be sure to eliminate anything that can distract you from your client while she is in your care.

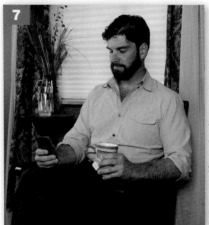

8 Before the client arrives, take a few quiet moments to prepare yourself with deep breathing, stretching, centering, and grounding.

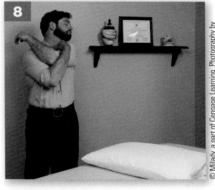

Greet Client

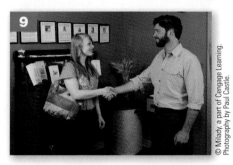

© Milady, a part of Cengage Learning. Photography by Paul Castle.

9 If this is the client's first visit, be ready to greet the client on time and introduce yourself with a handshake. In many places of business, the practitioner is addressed by their first name. For example, when introducing yourself to a new client, you might say, "Good morning, Mrs. Mason, I'm James. I'll be working with you today." You do not address the client by first name unless it is customary to do so or if the client requests that you do so.

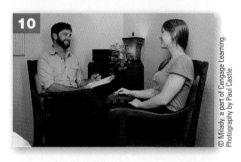

© Milady, a part of Cengage Learning. Photography by Paul Castle.

10 Perform a short consultation to determine the client's needs and determine any contraindications (see Box 4.1 for additional information on contraindications). Have the client fill out a client information sheet first, if applicable, and review it with the client to obtain more direct information. This is the time to observe the client's physical condition and determine which benefits might be derived from the massage or whether the client should be referred to another health care professional. If you are seeing a returning client, ask if there have been any changes since their last treatment. Determine a course of action for the treatment, and briefly explain your plan to the client.

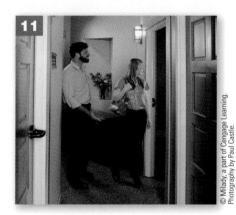

© Milady, a part of Cengage Learning. Photography by Paul Castle.

11 Put first-time clients at ease by touring the facility.

12 Escort the client to the massage area and prepare the table with fresh linens. Most practitioners prefer to spread the linens on the table in the presence of the client as an assurance that clean, fresh linens are used.

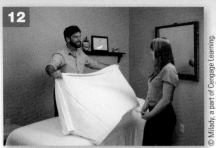

13 Explain to the client the preparation procedures regarding disrobing, getting on the table in a face-up position, and covering themselves with the top cover.

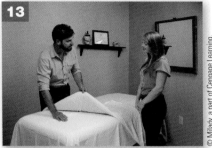

14 While the client is disrobing and getting on the table, the practitioner thoroughly washes their hands following the proper hand washing procedure. It is preferable to use warm water, pump soap and a clean and disinfected nail brush to wash under the free edge, and along the nail folds of the fingernails. Use a clean cloth or paper towel, according to the workplace policies, to dry the hands. Use that towel to turn off the faucet, and to open and/or close any doors between the sink and the treatment room. This prevents contamination and shows the client that the practitioner is considerate of their well-being.

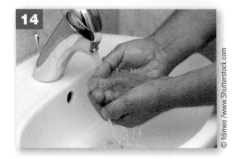

15 If the client has mobility impairments, it may be helpful to assist the client onto the massage table and into a supine (face-up) position to begin the massage.

16 Drape the client appropriately and provide extra support (pillows or bolsters) under the knees or head, if necessary.

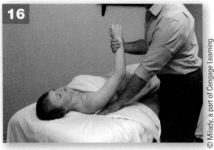

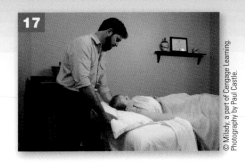

© Milady, a part of Cengage Learning. Photography by Paul Castle.

17 Attend to the client's comfort:

17a Ask whether the client is warm enough. Adjust the room temperature or provide an extra blanket if necessary.

17b Adjust pillows or bolsters so that the client is comfortable on the table.

17c Encourage the client to speak up at any time she feels discomfort of any kind so that adjustments can be made.

17d Observe the client throughout the treatment for any signs of discomfort and ask for feedback if any such signs are noted.

There are many possibilities for varying massage techniques for different clients. Every massage is unique, depending on the needs of the client and the practitioner's choices of the combination of massage techniques used during the session.

The following massage procedures will help you become more proficient and creative.

CONTRAINDICATIONS

It is the responsibility of the massage therapist to be aware of not only the benefits and indications for applying therapeutic massage techniques but also the contraindications and endangerment areas, to provide a positive and beneficial experience for the client.

A **contraindication** is any physical, emotional, or mental condition that could cause a particular massage treatment to be unsafe or detrimental to the client's well-being. Simply stated, a contraindication is a medical reason not to massage.

When there is doubt on the part of the practitioner as to whether to give a massage in the presence of a questionable condition, the client should be referred to her primary health care provider and obtain the physician's recommendations in writing. If the client does not have a primary physician, the practitioner may recommend an appropriate health care professional known to be familiar with and supportive of the practice of massage therapy.

Contraindications can be absolute, regional, or conditional:

☐ Absolute – meaning that massage should not be given until the condition subsides

☐ Regional or partial – meaning that massage is prohibited on a portion of the body because of a local condition

☐ Conditional – meaning there are health concerns for which certain massage techniques are not used because they could have adverse effects, whereas other techniques would be beneficial.

Careful questioning about the client's condition is essential during the consultation in determining whether any of the contraindications exist. Refer to *Theory & Practice of Therapeutic Massage* for more information on these contraindications.

- **Abnormal body temperature**. Massage is contraindicated when the client has a fever.
- **Acute infectious disease**. Examples include typhoid, diphtheria, severe colds, influenza, and similar illness preclude massage.
- **Inflammation**. There are numerous types of inflammations. When there is acute inflammation in a particular area of the body, massage is inadvisable because it could further irritate the area or intensify the inflammation.
  - *Inflammation from tissue damage*. Area becomes swollen and discolored.
  - *Inflammation from bacterial infestation*. Pus or pus pocket formed.

- *Osteoporosis*. Leads to deterioration of bone; symptoms include frailty and stooped shoulders.
- *Varicose veins*. A condition in which the valves in the veins break down because of back pressure in the circulatory system.
- *Phlebitis*. Inflammation of a vein accompanied by pain and swelling.
- *Postsurgical*. Obtain physician's permission. Do not massage over fresh incisions.
- *Aneurosa or aneurysm*. A local distention or ballooning of an artery due to a weakening wall.
- *Hematoma*. A mass of blood trapped in some tissue or cavity of the body and is the result of internal bleeding.
  - *Contusions or bruise*. A common type of hematoma that is generally not too serious.
- *Edema*. A circulatory abnormality that generally appears as puffiness or swelling in the extremities but is sometimes more widespread.
- *Lymphedema*. An accumulation of interstitial fluid, or swelling, in the soft tissues caused by inflammation, blockage, or removal of the lymph channels.

- **High blood pressure**.
- **Cancer**. Because massage enhances circulation, the application of massage must be modified when working with cancer patients.
- **Chronic fatigue**.
- **Intoxication**.
- **Psychosis**.
- **Medication and drugs**. All medications used by a client should be listed on the intake form.
- **Pregnancy**. It is best to postpone the first prenatal massage until after the twelfth week of the pregnancy. Obtain a release from the client's doctor.
- **Skin problems**:

• *Acne*	• *Impetigo*	• *Skin cancer*
• *Boils*	• *Inflammation*	• *Skin tags*
• *Broken vessels*	• *Lacerations*	• *Sores*
• *Bruises*	• *Lumps*	• *Stings and bites*
• *Burns and Blisters*	• *Rashes*	• *Tumor*
• *Carbuncles*	• *Scaly Spots*	• *Warts*
• *Hypersensitive skin*	• *Scratches*	• *Wounds*

- **Hernia or rupture**. A protrusion of an organ or part of an organ.
- **Frail elderly people**.
- **Scoliosis or crooked spine**.
- **Severe asthma**.
- **Diabetes**.
- **Any type of heart, lung, or kidney diseases**.

PERFORMANCE RUBRICS

Pre-Service Procedure

Rubrics are used in education for organizing and interpreting data gathered from observations of student performance. It is a clearly developed scoring document used to differentiate between levels of development in a specific skill performance or behavior. Rubrics are provided in this supplement for use as either a self-assessment tool to aid the student in behavior development or as an educator assessment tool to determine competence. Space is provided to record steps needed for further growth and improvement.

Performance is evaluated according to the following scale:

1 **Development Opportunity**: There is little or no evidence of competency; Assistance is needed; Performance includes multiple errors.

2 **Fundamental**: There is beginning evidence of competency; Task is completed alone; Performance includes few errors.

3 **Competent**: There is detailed and consistent evidence of competency; Task is completed alone; Performance includes rare errors.

4 **Strength**: There is detailed evidence of highly creative, inventive, mature presence of competency. Space is provided for comments to assist you in improving your performance and achieving a higher rating.

PERFORMANCE ASSESSED	1	2	3	4	IMPROVEMENT PLAN
Procedure					
1. Prepared the facility in regards to cleanliness and temperature.					
2. Reviewed client schedule to determine and collect all necessary materials and products needed for the day.					
3. Checked and replenished linens.					
4. Selected appropriate lubricants in proper dispenser containers.					
5. Reviewed client files of returning clients.					
6–7. Took care of personal needs before client arrived. Turned off cell phone, pager, or PDA.					
8. Took time to center and ground before client arrived.					
9. Greeted client in a professional manner.					
10. Performed a short consultation to determine a course of action for the massage.					
11. Toured the facility with the client.					
12. Prepared the table with fresh linens.					
13. Explained to the client the procedure for disrobing and getting on the table.					

PERFORMANCE ASSESSED	1	2	3	4	IMPROVEMENT PLAN
14. While the client was getting on the table the practitioner thoroughly washed their hands. Dried their hands with a paper towel and used that paper towel to turn off the faucet and to hold door knobs when opening and closing doors on the way to the massage room.					
15. Assisted any client with mobility impairments or other concerns onto the massage table in a supine position.					
16. Draped the client appropriately.					
17. Attended to client's comfort.					

Notes

Notes

Basic General Massage

The General Body Massage routine is simplified and flexible in that some steps can be omitted and others included. The General Body Massage routine is a basic routine and designed as an introductory massage for both the student and the client. It begins with the hand and arm, the least vulnerable and most safely accessible area of the body. The General Body Massage also does not include the face and head so that mussing the hair and makeup are not an issue. Students should follow the instructor's directions. The main objective is to give a beneficial and relaxing massage that is suited to the client's desires and needs.

Order of Treatment

The following procedure is suggested for a basic relaxing massage. However, it can be varied to suit the convenience of the practitioner and the needs of the client. Before beginning the massage, take a few deep, relaxing breaths to be more centered and grounded.

1. Begin with the hands and arms, right then left.

2. Proceed to the front of the legs and feet, left then right.

3. Continue movements over the abdomen, chest, and neck.

4. The client will turn over to assume a prone (face-down) position.

5. Begin with the back of the legs, right then left.

6. Finish the massage with the back of the body.

7. Following the massage, the client should be allowed to rest for a short period and then be assisted from the table.

General Arm Massage

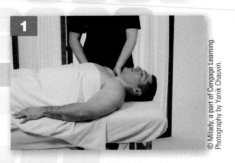

© Milady, a part of Cengage Learning. Photography by Yanik Chauvin.

1 Undrape an arm in preparation for massage.

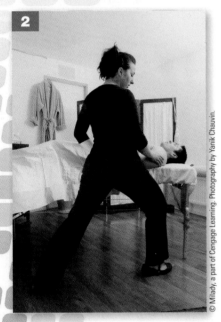

© Milady, a part of Cengage Learning. Photography by Yanik Chauvin.

2 Apply the lubricant with a light, smooth effleurage stroke from the shoulder to the hand. A light stroke allows the lubricant to be distributed along the entire length of the arm. Proper body mechanics reduces fatigue and allows for mobility and power when performing massage.

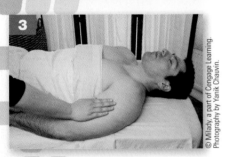

© Milady, a part of Cengage Learning. Photography by Yanik Chauvin.

3 Apply effleurage to the arm three to five times. Beginning at the wrist, apply a gliding stroke up the arm and over the shoulder with a firm pressure. Allow the hand to conform to the shape of the arm as it glides over the forearm, elbow, upper arm, and shoulder. Reduce the pressure and continue with a light effleurage stroke back down the arm to the wrist.

4 Apply effleurage to both the anterior and posterior aspects of the arm.

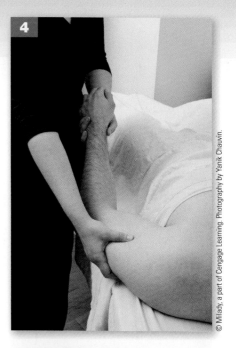

5 Knead the arm from the shoulder to the wrist. Beginning as close to the shoulder as possible, using both hands, one on each side of the arm, apply petrissage, directing each stroke towards the heart while working down the arm. The hands can work in unison or alternately.

6 Apply effleurage from the wrist to the shoulder. Repeat steps 3 and 4 above.

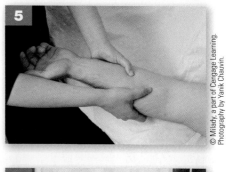

7 Roll the arm from the elbow to the wrist. Bend the arm at the elbow and rest the elbow on the table with the hand pointing to the ceiling. With one hand on each side of the forearm, briskly roll the forearm from the elbow to the wrist.

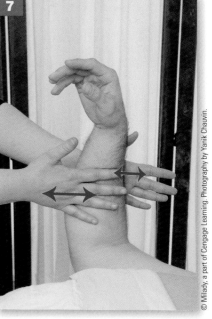

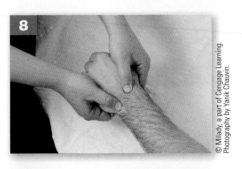

8 Apply petrissage to the carpals and metacarpals on the back of the hand.

© Milady, a part of Cengage Learning. Photography by Yanik Chauvin.

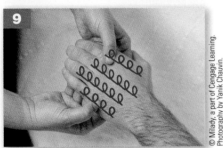

9 Apply friction movements to the back of the hand.

© Milady, a part of Cengage Learning. Photography by Yanik Chauvin.

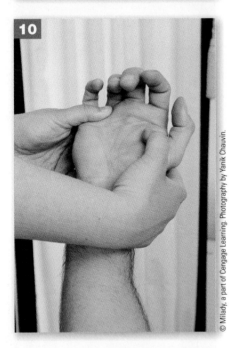

10 Turn the hand over and thoroughly massage the palm of the hand with your thumbs.

© Milady, a part of Cengage Learning. Photography by Yanik Chauvin.

11 Stabilize the client's hand with one hand and knead and circumduct each finger while applying a slight traction.

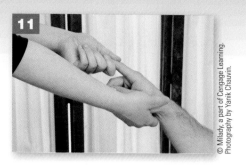

© Milady, a part of Cengage Learning. Photography by Yanik Chauvin.

12 Flex all four fingers together. Grasp the client's hand to stabilize it with your other hand and flex the fingers.

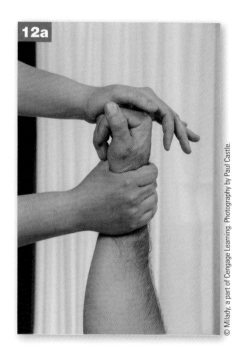

© Milady, a part of Cengage Learning. Photography by Paul Castle.

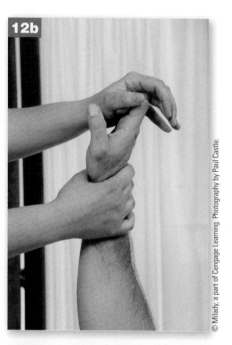

© Milady, a part of Cengage Learning. Photography by Paul Castle.

13 Extend and circumduct all four fingers in unison.

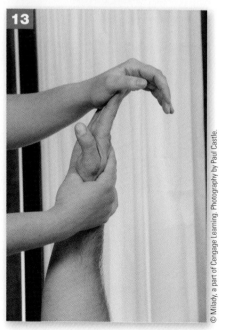

© Milady, a part of Cengage Learning. Photography by Paul Castle.

General Arm Massage continued

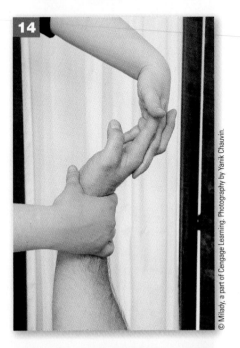

© Milady, a part of Cengage Learning. Photography by Yanik Chauvin.

14 Move the stabilizing hand to the forearm and flex, extend, and circumduct the client's wrist.

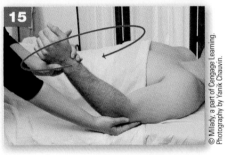

© Milady, a part of Cengage Learning. Photography by Yanik Chauvin.

15 Stabilize the elbow on the table and rotate and circumduct the forearm.

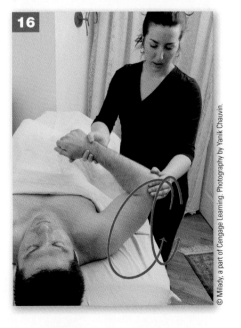

© Milady, a part of Cengage Learning. Photography by Yanik Chauvin.

16 Hold the client's elbow and wrist and move the arm to flex and rotate the shoulder.

17 Straighten the elbow and circumduct the shoulder.

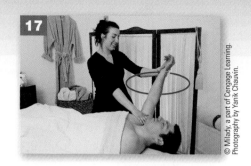

18 Apply effleurage to the arm. Repeat steps 3 and 4.

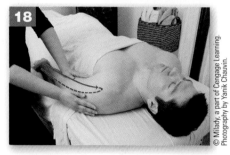

19 Apply feather (nerve) strokes from the shoulder to the fingertips and re-drape the arm.

20 Move to the other arm and repeat the sequence.

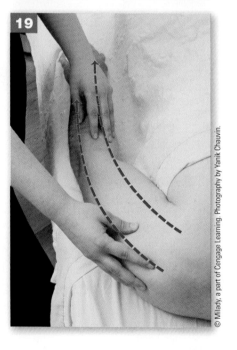

General Arm Massage

Rubrics are used in education for organizing and interpreting data gathered from observations of student performance. It is a clearly developed scoring document used to differentiate between levels of development in a specific skill performance or behavior. Rubrics are provided in this supplement for use as either a self-assessment tool to aid the student in behavior development or as an educator assessment tool to determine competence. Space is provided to record steps needed for further growth and improvement.

Performance is evaluated according to the following scale:

1 **Development Opportunity:** There is little or no evidence of competency; Assistance is needed; Performance includes multiple errors.

2 **Fundamental:** There is beginning evidence of competency; Task is completed alone; Performance includes few errors.

3 **Competent:** There is detailed and consistent evidence of competency; Task is completed alone; Performance includes rare errors.

4 **Strength:** There is detailed evidence of highly creative, inventive, mature presence of competency. Space is provided for comments to assist you in improving your performance and achieving a higher rating.

PERFORMANCE ASSESSED	1	2	3	4	IMPROVEMENT PLAN
Procedure					
1. Undraped the arm.					
2. Applied the lubricant with long effleurage stroke.					
3. Applied effleurage to the entire arm 3–5 times.					
4. Applied effleurage to both anterior and posterior aspects of the arm.					
5. Kneaded the arm from shoulder to wrist.					
6. Applied effleurage from wrist to shoulder 3–5 times.					
7. Rolled the arm from elbow to wrist.					
8. Applied petrissage to the back of the hand.					
9. Applied friction to the back of the hand.					
10. Massaged the palm of the hand with the thumbs.					
11. Applied kneading and circumduction to each finger.					
12. Applied flexion to all the fingers.					
13. Applied extension and circumduction to all the fingers in unison.					

PERFORMANCE ASSESSED	1	2	3	4	IMPROVEMENT PLAN
14. Applied flexion, extension, and circumduction to the wrist.					
15. Applied rotation and circumduction to the forearm.					
16. Applied flexion and rotation to the shoulder.					
17. Straightened the elbow and circumducted the shoulder.					
18. Applied effleurage to the entire arm 3–5 times.					
19. Applied feather strokes to the arm.					
20a. Re-draped the arm.					
20b. Repeated the massage sequence on the other arm.					

Notes

General Massage for the Foot and Leg

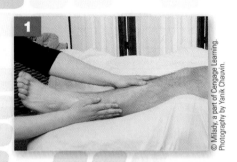

© Milady, a part of Cengage Learning. Photography by Yanik Chauvin.

1 Undrape one leg (on the same side of the body as the arm that was just completed) in preparation for massage.

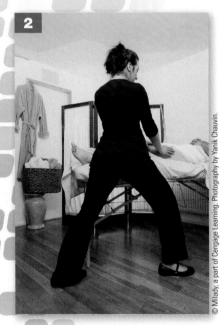

© Milady, a part of Cengage Learning. Photography by Yanik Chauvin.

2 Apply lubricant with a light, smooth effleurage stroke from the foot to the hip and back to the foot. The leg is the longest part of the body so it is important to practice proper body mechanics. A wide archer's stance allows the practitioner to massage the entire length of the leg.

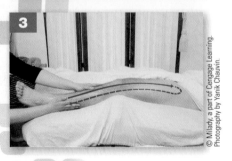

© Milady, a part of Cengage Learning. Photography by Yanik Chauvin.

3 Apply effleurage to the leg. Begin at the ankle with both hands covering the anterior surface applying a gentle, firm pressure, gliding up the leg. Allow flexibility in the hands to follow the contours of the leg, leading slightly with the lateral hand as it glides up over the thigh nearly to the iliac crest. The medial hand glides two-thirds of the way over the thigh and then both hands reverse direction and with a lighter pressure, returning to the starting point near the ankle. Repeat the stroke three to five times.

4 Apply kneading to the top, bottom, and sides of the foot.

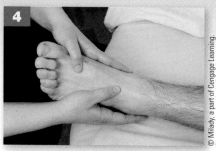

5 Continue kneading with warming, relaxing circles on the sides of the foot and ankle.

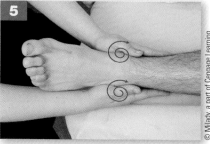

6 Apply circular friction between the tendons and other surfaces on the top and sides of the foot.

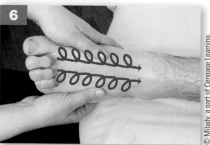

7 Knead and circumduct each toe between your thumb and fingers.

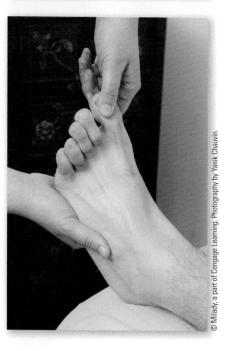

General Massage for the Foot and Leg continued

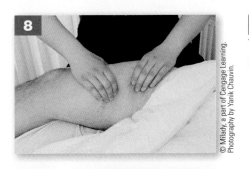

© Milady, a part of Cengage Learning. Photography by Yanik Chauvin.

8 Apply petrissage to the leg, beginning at the ankle and working up over the thigh and then back down to the ankle. It may require several passes to petrissage all the muscles of the thigh.

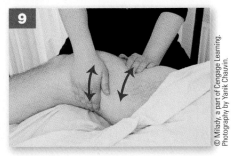

© Milady, a part of Cengage Learning. Photography by Yanik Chauvin.

9 Wring the anterior thigh and lower leg.

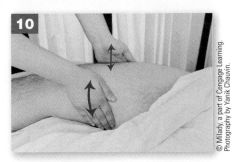

© Milady, a part of Cengage Learning. Photography by Yanik Chauvin.

10 Roll the muscles of the thigh.

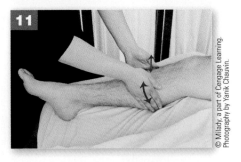

© Milady, a part of Cengage Learning. Photography by Yanik Chauvin.

11 Continue the rolling movement, working down the lower leg.

12 Repeat effleurage to the leg three to five times. Repeat step 3.

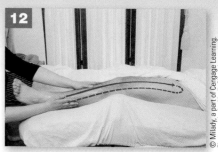

13 Apply joint movements to the foot; begin by dorsal flexing the foot and toes.

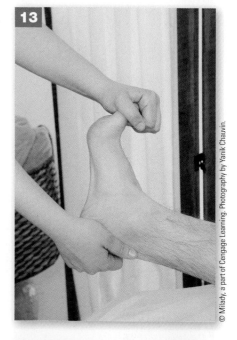

14 Continue joint movements by plantar flexing the foot and ankle.

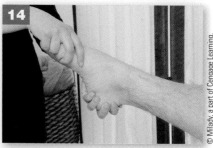

15 Stretch the Achilles tendon and muscles of the calf by dorsal flexing the foot and ankle with the knee extended.

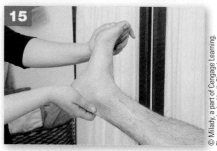

General Massage for the Foot and Leg continued

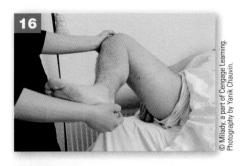

16 Flex the knee and hip and move the client's knee toward their chest. Be careful to maintain good draping while moving the leg.

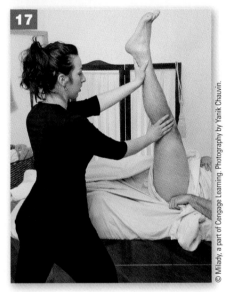

17 Extend the knee while keeping the hip flexed to stretch the hamstring muscles, and then return the leg to the table.

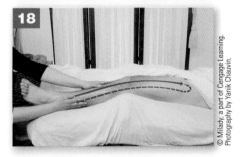

18 Apply effleurage again to the leg lightly three times.

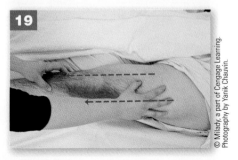

19 Apply feather (nerve) strokes and re-drape the leg.

20 Move to the other leg and complete the sequence.

General Massage for the Foot and Leg

Rubrics are used in education for organizing and interpreting data gathered from observations of student performance. It is a clearly developed scoring document used to differentiate between levels of development in a specific skill performance or behavior. Rubrics are provided in this supplement for use as either a self-assessment tool to aid the student in behavior development or as an educator assessment tool to determine competence. Space is provided to record steps needed for further growth and improvement.

Performance is evaluated according to the following scale:

1 **Development Opportunity:** There is little or no evidence of competency; Assistance is needed; Performance includes multiple errors.

2 **Fundamental:** There is beginning evidence of competency; Task is completed alone; Performance includes few errors.

3 **Competent:** There is detailed and consistent evidence of competency; Task is completed alone; Performance includes rare errors.

4 **Strength:** There is detailed evidence of highly creative, inventive, mature presence of competency. Space is provided for comments to assist you in improving your performance and achieving a higher rating.

PERFORMANCE ASSESSED	1	2	3	4	IMPROVEMENT PLAN
Procedure					
1. Undraped the leg.					
2. Applied the lubricant with a light effleurage stroke.					
3. Applied effleurage to the leg 3–5 times.					
4. Applied kneading to the top, bottom, and sides of the foot.					
5. Continued kneading with warming, relaxing circles on the sides of the foot and ankle.					
6. Applied circular friction between the tendons on the top and sides of the foot.					
7. Applied kneading and circumduction to the toes.					
8. Applied petrissage to the lower leg and thigh.					
9. Applied wringing to the thigh and lower leg.					
10. Applied rolling to the thigh.					
11. Continued the rolling movement, working down the lower leg.					
12. Applied effleurage to the leg 3–5 times.					
13. Applied joint movements to the foot; begun by dorsal flexing the foot and toes.					

PERFORMANCE ASSESSED	1	2	3	4	IMPROVEMENT PLAN
14. Continued joint movements by plantar flexing the foot.					
15. Stretched the Achilles tendon and calf muscles by dorsal flexing the foot and ankle.					
16. Applied joint movements to the knee and hip.					
17. Flexed the hip joint to stretch the hamstrings. Then returned the leg to the table.					
18. Applied effleurage 3–5 times.					
19. Applied feather strokes. Re-draped the leg.					
20. Completed the entire sequence on the other leg.					

Notes

_____

_____

_____

_____

_____

_____

_____

_____

General Massage for the Anterior Torso and Neck

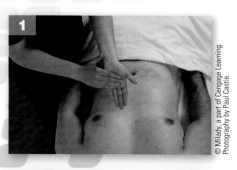

© Milady, a part of Cengage Learning. Photography by Paul Castle.

1 On a male client, undrape the torso to a level midway between the navel and the pubic bone to expose the abdomen.

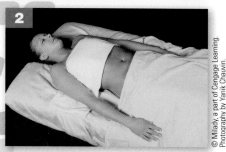

© Milady, a part of Cengage Learning. Photography by Yanik Chauvin.

2 On a female, use breast draping. Some of the following strokes can be modified to accommodate the breast drape.

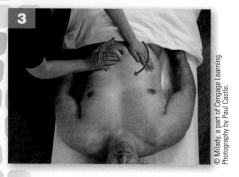

© Milady, a part of Cengage Learning. Photography by Paul Castle.

3 Standing on the left side of the client, apply circular effleurage on the abdomen in a clockwise direction, following the direction of the colon.

General Massage for the Anterior Torso and Neck continued

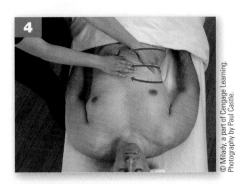

4 Apply deep gliding strokes to the opposite side of the body from near the table to the midline of the body (these repeated gliding strokes are commonly referred to as *shingles*). Begin the first stroke just inferior to the crest of the ilium. When the first stroke is near the midline, begin the next stroke with the other hand. Continue alternating hands, moving slowly up the body toward the axilla.

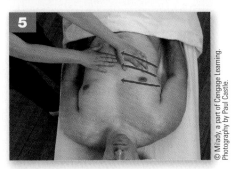

5 In the area of the ribs, flex the fingertips for a raking effect between the ribs. (When using breast draping, proceed up the side of the torso as far as the draping will allow and then back down to the hip.)

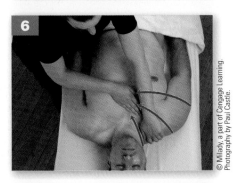

6 Continue the alternate-hand effleurage (shingles) to the axillary area, over the shoulder, and up the neck.

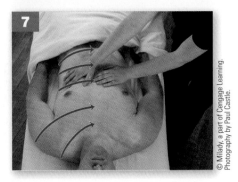

7 Switch sides of the table and continue the shingles stroke down the other side of the torso from the neck to the ilium and then back to the axillary area, once again raking over the ribs.

8 Apply petrissage to the pectoral area, first one side, and then the other. (Avoid breast tissue on women.)

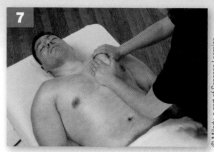

9 Move to the head of the table. Apply a long effleurage stroke, often referred to as a "caring stroke." The caring stroke covers the entire front of the torso and the neck. It is not possible to perform the caring stroke on a woman using breast draping. It begins at the sternal notch with a long effleurage stroke down the front of the chest and abdomen to the pubic bone.

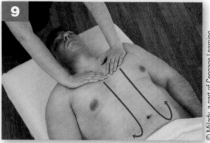

10 Without losing contact with the client, rotate your hands and continue gliding up the side of the torso to the axilla. Glide up, over, and around the shoulders and up the neck. Again, rotate your hands and return to the starting spot and repeat the caring stroke three to five times.

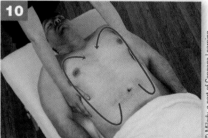

11 The caring stroke can be abbreviated when working on the neck or when using breast draping. From the head of the table, apply effleurage with both hands, beginning at the sternal notch and gliding out over the shoulders.

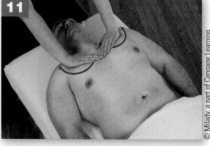

12 Continue to glide out over and around the shoulders.

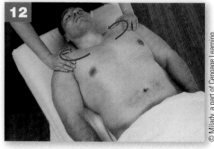

General Massage for the Anterior Torso and Neck continued

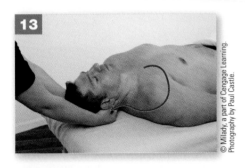

13 Continue to glide up the trapezius to the occipital ridge, rotate your hands, glide back down the neck to the starting position, and repeat the stroke three to five times.

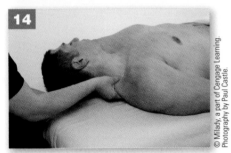

14 Turn the client's head to one side and apply petrissage to the back and sides of the neck and shoulders.

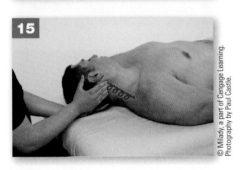

15 While the head is still turned to the side, apply circular friction along the occiput and down the side of the neck. Pay attention to any tight or congested areas. Repeat friction and kneading over those areas.

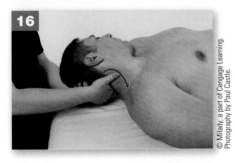

16 Apply deep gliding strokes from the occiput down the shoulders using the thumbs or fingertips. Use caution to not pull the hair on the back of the neck.

17 Turn the client's head to the other side and apply petrissage and circular friction to that side of the neck.

18 Apply deep gliding strokes from the occiput down the neck and shoulder.

19 Repeat effleurage over the shoulders, as in steps 11 through 13.

20 Re-drape the torso.

General Massage for the Anterior Torso and Neck

Rubrics are used in education for organizing and interpreting data gathered from observations of student performance. It is a clearly developed scoring document used to differentiate between levels of development in a specific skill performance or behavior. Rubrics are provided in this supplement for use as either a self-assessment tool to aid the student in behavior development or as an educator assessment tool to determine competence. Space is provided to record steps needed for further growth and improvement.

Performance is evaluated according to the following scale:

1 **Development Opportunity:** There is little or no evidence of competency; Assistance is needed; Performance includes multiple errors.

2 **Fundamental:** There is beginning evidence of competency; Task is completed alone; Performance includes few errors.

3 **Competent:** There is detailed and consistent evidence of competency; Task is completed alone; Performance includes rare errors.

4 **Strength:** There is detailed evidence of highly creative, inventive, mature presence of competency. Space is provided for comments to assist you in improving your performance and achieving a higher rating.

PERFORMANCE ASSESSED	1	2	3	4	IMPROVEMENT PLAN
Procedure					
1–2. Undraped the chest and abdomen of a male client. Note: if client was a female, used breast draping.					
3. While standing on the left side of the client, applied circular effleurage to the abdomen.					
4. Applied alternating-hand stroking (shingles) from the ilium to the axillary area.					
5. Flexed the fingertips and applied raking over the ribs.					
6. Continued the shingles movement over the shoulder and up the neck.					
7. Moved to the other side of the table and continued the shingles movement down the opposite side of the neck, over the shoulder, and down to the ilium, once again, raking over the ribs.					
8. Applied petrissage to the pectoral area, first one side then the other.					
9. Moved to the head of the table and applied the caring stroke beginning at the sternal notch with a long effleurage down over the chest and abdomen.					

PERFORMANCE ASSESSED	1	2	3	4	IMPROVEMENT PLAN
10. Continued the caring stroke out to the sides of the torso, up to the axilla, around the shoulders, and back to the starting point. Repeated the caring stroke three to five times.					
11. When using breast draping, abbreviated the caring stroke by beginning at the sternal notch, applied a bi-lateral effleurage stroke out toward the shoulders.					
12. Continued the effleurage stroke out over and around the shoulders.					
13. Continued the bilateral effleurage stroke up the trapezius to the occipital ridge, and rotated the hands to glide down the sides of the neck to the starting point. Repeated the stroke three to five times.					
14. Turned the client's head to one side and applied petrissage to the neck and shoulders.					
15. While the head was still turned, applied circular friction along the occiput and down the side of the neck.					
16. Applied deep gliding strokes from the occiput down the neck and shoulders.					
17. Turned the client's head the opposite direction and applied petrissage and friction to the muscles of the neck and shoulders.					
18. Applied deep gliding strokes from the occiput, down the neck, and shoulders.					
19. Returned the client's head to neutral and repeated bilateral effleurage around the shoulders and up the trapezius to the occiput.					
20. Re-draped the torso.					

Changing Position from Supine to Prone

Overview

When it is time for the client to turn over to a prone, face-down position, maintain proper draping to prevent exposure while the client is turning. If using a face rest, put it in place at the head of the table.

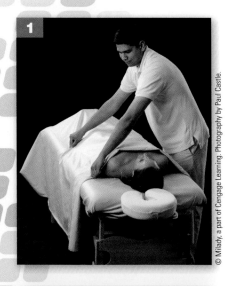

1 With the client supine, straighten the top cover and hold it in place in three places by leaning against the table with the thighs, and reaching across the client to grasp the top cover at the level of the client's shoulder with one hand and their mid-thigh with the other.

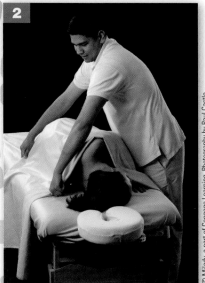

2 Allow some slack in the top cover. Instruct the client to roll over by first facing you, and then continuing to roll onto their stomach. Hold the top sheet in place as the client roles onto their stomach under the cover.

Changing Position from Supine to Prone continued

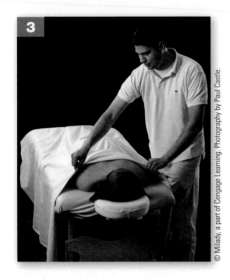

© Milady, a part of Cengage Learning. Photography by Paul Castle.

3 Instruct the client to move up on the table until their face is aligned in the face rest. If necessary, adjust the face cradle for comfort.

4 Readjust the top cover.

PERFORMANCE RUBRICS

Changing Position from Supine to Prone

Rubrics are used in education for organizing and interpreting data gathered from observations of student performance. It is a clearly developed scoring document used to differentiate between levels of development in a specific skill performance or behavior. Rubrics are provided in this supplement for use as either a self-assessment tool to aid the student in behavior development or as an educator assessment tool to determine competence. Space is provided to record steps needed for further growth and improvement.

Performance is evaluated according to the following scale:

1 Development Opportunity: There is little or no evidence of competency; Assistance is needed; Performance includes multiple errors.

2 Fundamental: There is beginning evidence of competency; Task is completed alone; Performance includes few errors.

3 Competent: There is detailed and consistent evidence of competency; Task is completed alone; Performance includes rare errors.

4 Strength: There is detailed evidence of highly creative, inventive, mature presence of competency. Space is provided for comments to assist you in improving your performance and achieving a higher rating.

PERFORMANCE ASSESSED	1	2	3	4	IMPROVEMENT PLAN
Procedure					
1. Positioned the face rest at the head of the massage table. Positioned the top cover and held it in place.					
2. Instructed the client to role towards you and onto their stomach.					
3. Instructed the client to move up on the table and position their face comfortably in the face rest.					
4. Re-adjusted the top cover.					

General Massage for the Back of the Legs

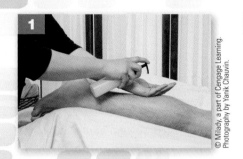

© Milady, a part of Cengage Learning. Photography by Yanik Chauvin.

1 Undrape one leg and apply lubricant with a light effleurage stroke to the entire posterior leg.

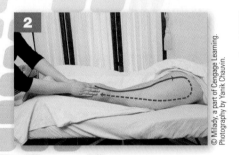

© Milady, a part of Cengage Learning. Photography by Yanik Chauvin.

2 Move the leg closer to the edge of the table and apply effleurage from the heel to the hip three times. Using both hands to apply effleurage, lead with the lateral hand gliding up and over the gluteal muscle while the medial hand proceeds only to the gluteal crease before returning to the ankle with a much lighter stroke. More pressure is applied on the stroke from the foot to the hip (distal to proximal) with a light contact from the hip to the foot.

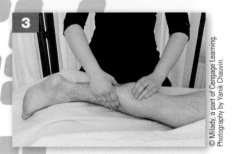

© Milady, a part of Cengage Learning. Photography by Yanik Chauvin.

3 Apply petrissage to the leg from the hips to the heels.

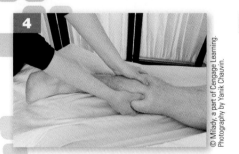

© Milady, a part of Cengage Learning. Photography by Yanik Chauvin.

4 Apply fulling to the posterior thigh and lower leg.

5 Apply wringing to the posterior thigh and leg.

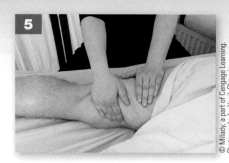

© Milady, a part of Cengage Learning.
Photography by Yanik Chauvin.

6 Apply effleurage to the leg three to five times.

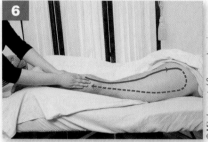

© Milady, a part of Cengage Learning.
Photography by Yanik Chauvin.

7 Apply nerve strokes to the posterior leg and re-drape.

8 Repeat the sequence to the other leg or move on to the back.

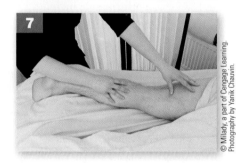

© Milady, a part of Cengage Learning.
Photography by Yanik Chauvin.

General Massage for the Back of the Legs

Rubrics are used in education for organizing and interpreting data gathered from observations of student performance. It is a clearly developed scoring document used to differentiate between levels of development in a specific skill performance or behavior. Rubrics are provided in this supplement for use as either a self-assessment tool to aid the student in behavior development or as an educator assessment tool to determine competence. Space is provided to record steps needed for further growth and improvement.

Performance is evaluated according to the following scale:

1 **Development Opportunity:** There is little or no evidence of competency; Assistance is needed; Performance includes multiple errors.

2 **Fundamental:** There is beginning evidence of competency; Task is completed alone; Performance includes few errors.

3 **Competent:** There is detailed and consistent evidence of competency; Task is completed alone; Performance includes rare errors.

4 **Strength:** There is detailed evidence of highly creative, inventive, mature presence of competency. Space is provided for comments to assist you in improving your performance and achieving a higher rating.

PERFORMANCE ASSESSED	1	2	3	4	IMPROVEMENT PLAN
Procedure					
1. Undraped the posterior leg and applied lubricant to the entire posterior leg.					
2. Applied effleurage from the heel to the hip three to five times.					
3. Applied petrissage from the hip to the heel.					
4. Applied fulling to the posterior thigh and leg.					
5. Applied wringing to the posterior leg and thigh.					
6. Applied effleurage to the posterior leg three to five times.					
7a. Applied nerve strokes to the posterior leg.					
7b. Re-draped the posterior leg.					
8. Repeated sequence to the other leg.					

General Massage for the Back of the Body

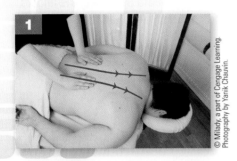

1 Undrape the back down to the level of the gluteal cleft and apply lubricant to the entire back with long, even gliding strokes.

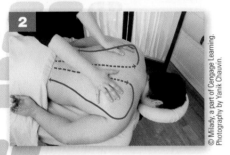

2 Standing at the side of the client, apply effleurage to the back five times, beginning on the low back and going up along the muscles on each side of the spine. Then, continue the stroke out over the shoulders and down on the side of the back.

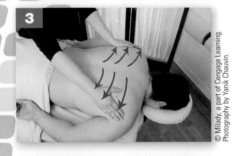

3 Place the hands flat on each side of the spine at the level of the scapulas and apply deep gliding strokes from the midline of the back outward toward the shoulders.

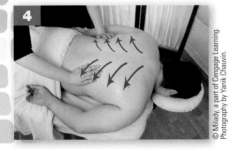

4 Continue step 3 down along each side of the spine to cover the entire back (fan stroke).

General Massage for the Back of the Body continued

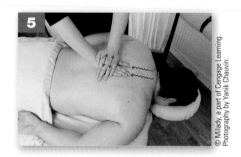

5 Vibrate along each side of the vertebral column from the neck to the sacrum. Apply vibration movements along each vertebra by placing the fingers of one hand on each side of the spinous process and the other hand on top. Vibrate back and forth as you move down along the spine.

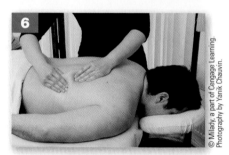

6 Apply petrissage on the entire side of the back that is opposite where you are standing. This may require several passes.

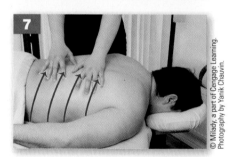

7 Apply alternate hand, deep gliding strokes on the far side of the torso from the table to the center of the back (shingles) from the hips to the shoulders. In the area of the ribs, flex the tips of your fingers for a raking effect.

8 Move to the other side of the table and repeat steps 6 and 7.

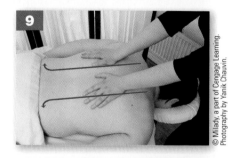

9 From the head of the table, apply effleurage to cover the entire back three to five times. This stroke is commonly called a *caring stroke*. Beginning at the back of the neck, stroke down along the length of the muscles on the side of the spine to the ilium.

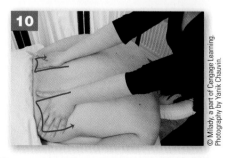

10 Continue the effleurage stroke around to the side of the body and up the sides.

11 The caring stroke continues around and over the shoulders, up to the neck, and then repeats.

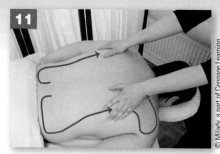

12 Move to the side of the table and apply light hacking movements along the muscles on the side of the spine, between the shoulders, over the gluteal muscles, and the back of the legs. Avoid percussion over the kidney area.

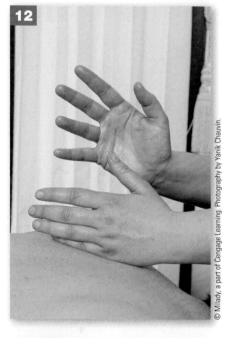

13 From the side of the table, lightly apply effleurage to the back several times.

14 Apply nerve strokes to the entire back, from the head all the way to the feet.

15 Re-drape the back and complete the massage.

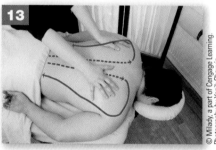

General Massage for the Back of the Body

Rubrics are used in education for organizing and interpreting data gathered from observations of student performance. It is a clearly developed scoring document used to differentiate between levels of development in a specific skill performance or behavior. Rubrics are provided in this supplement for use as either a self-assessment tool to aid the student in behavior development or as an educator assessment tool to determine competence. Space is provided to record steps needed for further growth and improvement.

Performance is evaluated according to the following scale:

1 Development Opportunity: There is little or no evidence of competency; Assistance is needed; Performance includes multiple errors.

2 Fundamental: There is beginning evidence of competency; Task is completed alone; Performance includes few errors.

3 Competent: There is detailed and consistent evidence of competency; Task is completed alone; Performance includes rare errors.

4 Strength: There is detailed evidence of highly creative, inventive, mature presence of competency. Space is provided for comments to assist you in improving your performance and achieving a higher rating.

PERFORMANCE ASSESSED	1	2	3	4	IMPROVEMENT PLAN
Procedure					
1. Undraped the back and applied lubricant to the entire back.					
2. Stood at the side of the table and applied effleurage up the back, over the shoulders, and down the side of the client's back.					
3. Applied gliding strokes from the midline of the back to the sides (fan strokes).					
4. Continued fan strokes from the scapulas down the entire back.					
5. Applied vibration to the muscles along the vertebra from the neck to the sacrum.					
6. Applied petrissage to the entire side of the back.					
7. Applied deep gliding strokes on the far side of the torso from the table to the midline of the back (shingles). Continued "shingles" strokes from the ilium, up the side, over the shoulder, and up the neck.					
8. Moved to the other side of the table and applied petrissage and shingles to the other side of the back.					
9. Moved to the head of the table and applied effleurage to the entire back, beginning at the back of the neck stroke down the muscles on each side of the spine to the ilium.					

PERFORMANCE ASSESSED	1	2	3	4	IMPROVEMENT PLAN
10. Continued the effleurage stroke around to the side of the body and up the sides.					
11. Continued the caring stroke around and over the shoulders up to the neck and then repeated this motion three to five times.					
12. Applied hacking to the back. Avoided percussion over the kidney area.					
13. From the side of the table, applied effleurage to the back.					
14. Applied nerve strokes from the head to the feet.					
15. Re-draped the back.					

Notes

Post-Service: Completing the General Massage Session

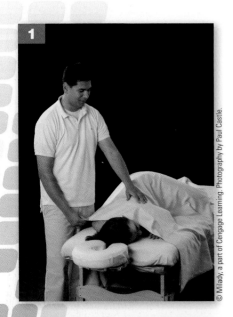

1 After completing the final strokes, maintain light contact. Allow the client a few moments to savor the deep relaxation as she returns to a more conscious state. Adjust the draping, and suggest that the client turn onto her side.

2 When it is time to get up, instruct the client to put her legs over the edge of the table and push herself into a sitting position with her arm.

3 As she sits up, she can secure the wrap. You may assist the client by placing a hand under her shoulder and lifting her into a sitting position.

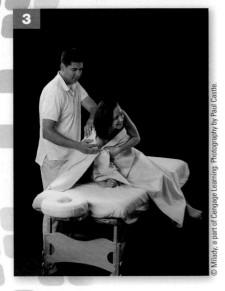

4 Suggest supplementary services and answer any questions that the client might have.

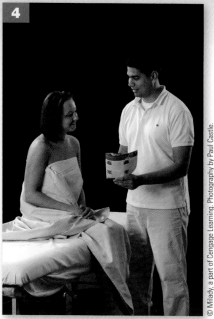

5 When she is totally awake and reoriented, assist the client off the table and direct her to the dressing area. A sturdy step stool may be used if the table is tall.

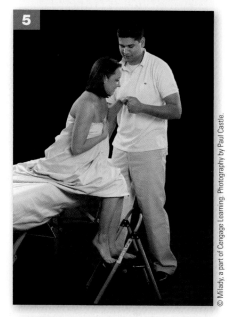

6 After the client is dressed, collect your fees and set up the next appointment.

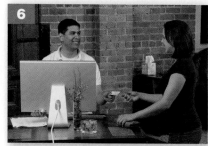

Post-Service: Completing the General Massage Session continued

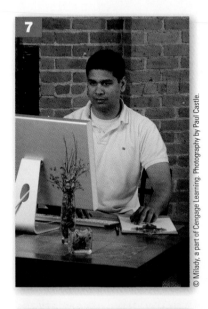
© Milady, a part of Cengage Learning. Photography by Paul Castle.

7 | As soon as the client leaves, complete the client's record or SOAP notes.

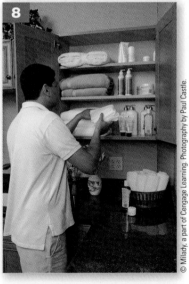
© Milady, a part of Cengage Learning. Photography by Paul Castle.

8 | Place supplies in their proper place; discard used items.

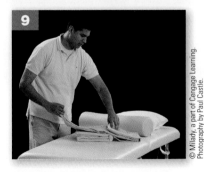
© Milady, a part of Cengage Learning. Photography by Paul Castle.

9 | See that all equipment and items, including the massage table, are properly prepared before the next client arrives.

Post-Service: Completing the General Massage Session

Rubrics are used in education for organizing and interpreting data gathered from observations of student performance. It is a clearly developed scoring document used to differentiate between levels of development in a specific skill performance or behavior. Rubrics are provided in this supplement for use as either a self-assessment tool to aid the student in behavior development or as an educator assessment tool to determine competence. Space is provided to record steps needed for further growth and improvement.

Performance is evaluated according to the following scale:

1 **Development Opportunity:** There is little or no evidence of competency; Assistance is needed; Performance includes multiple errors.

2 **Fundamental:** There is beginning evidence of competency; Task is completed alone; Performance includes few errors.

3 **Competent:** There is detailed and consistent evidence of competency; Task is completed alone; Performance includes rare errors.

4 **Strength:** There is detailed evidence of highly creative, inventive, mature presence of competency. Space is provided for comments to assist you in improving your performance and achieving a higher rating.

PERFORMANCE ASSESSED	1	2	3	4	IMPROVEMENT PLAN
Procedure					
1a. Maintained light contact after completing final feather (nerve) strokes.					
1b. Adjusted the draping, and suggested that the client turn onto their side. Optional: provided a pillow for their head.					
2–3. After a few minutes of rest, helped client into a sitting position while securing wrap to assure modesty.					
4. Suggested supplementary services and answered any questions the client may have.					
5. Assisted the client off the table and directed them to the dressing area.					
6. Collected fees and set up the next appointment.					
7. Completed client records or SOAP notes.					
8. Placed supplies and products in proper places. Discarded used, disposable items.					
9. Prepared the premises for the next client.					

Notes

Full Body Relaxation Massage

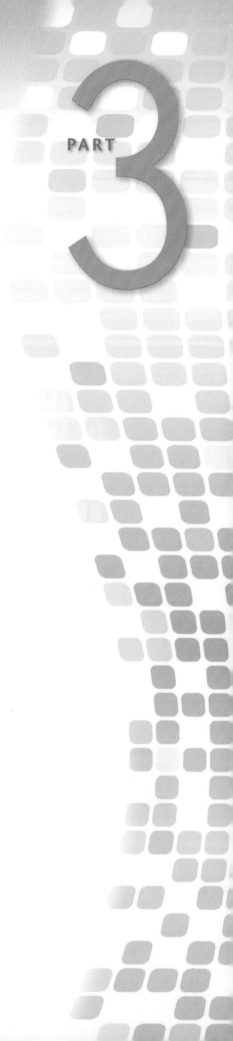

Massage, like any other skill, requires practice and patience to learn the basics, build speed, and develop new techniques. Each time you give a massage, you will find yourself becoming more innovative and more confident of your techniques. By the time you have learned the General Swedish Massage, you should be familiar with most of the terms for the various movements used in basic body massage.

The Full Body Relaxation Massage incorporates the sequencing and massage movements of the General Swedish Massage and introduces additional techniques to help you increase efficiency, remember the sequence of movements, and readily identify the movements and the parts of the anatomy by their proper names. While doing massage, pay attention to your hand positions, your stance, and how you move when delivering the strokes. Always maintain good body and table mechanics. Become more aware of the qualities of the tissues as you glide over and massage into each area of the body. Be sensitive to the different textures of the skin, the underlying fascia, and muscles. Begin to sense areas of tension and congestion where it might be appropriate to linger or use additional techniques in that area.

This Relaxation Massage procedure enables you to review what you have learned and allows even more creativity in varying massage routines. Before beginning the massage, concentrate on projecting the manner, attitude, and appearance of the professional massage practitioner. Read directions carefully for each step. After you have learned how to give a complete massage correctly and efficiently, you will no longer need to refer to your notes, illustrations, or written guides. Your aim is to be able to give the complete massage knowledgeably and professionally.

Massage the Face

Overview

The following procedure is a generalized massage routine designed as a relaxing full-body massage. It is only a guideline, and you can vary or alter it to fit the needs of each individual client and situation.

The client is positioned face up (supine) on the massage table with a bolster under her knees to relieve any tension in the lower back. The head is resting on the table in a neutral position unless the client exhibits a severe head-forward position, in which case a folded towel or a small pillow can be placed under her head. The practitioner should be standing or seated above the client's head, facing the client.

Face massage can be done as the opening procedure of the massage, or for various reasons, massaging the face may be left out of the massage routine. If the client is wearing makeup, she might choose to not have a face massage, or to remove the makeup herself before the session, or to proceed with the massage over the makeup. For sanitary reasons, when a face massage is included, it is usually at the beginning of the massage when the practitioner's hands have been freshly washed. Inform the client that very little lubricant is used, if any at all, for the face massage.

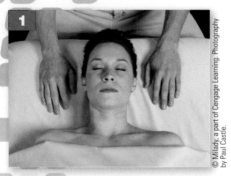
© Milady, a part of Cengage Learning. Photography by Paul Castle.

1   If the massage begins with the face, once both client and therapist are in place, the therapist can take a moment to quiet his thoughts, center and ground himself, and create intention before making initial contact with the client.

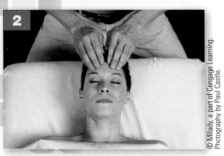
© Milady, a part of Cengage Learning. Photography by Paul Castle.

2   You can make the initial contact by lightly placing the finger pads of both hands on the frontal eminence of the forehead and resting them there for several seconds. This is a good time to focus on the connection with the client. After a short time, a light pulse may be noted under the fingertips, indicating relaxation of the frontalis muscle and circulation in the area. The practitioner might prefer to make first contact by placing the hands on the client's shoulders if the face is not being massage.

3 After a moment or when the pulse is noted, gently draw the fingers toward the hairline, gently stretching the frontalis muscle.

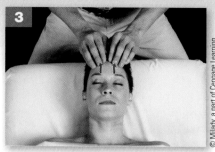

4 Place thumbs from both hands in the center of the forehead at the hairline. With slight pressure, glide the thumbs along the hairline to the temples and conclude with gentle circular friction applied with the fingertips at the temples. Return the thumb to the midline, about a finger's-width inferior to the first gliding stroke and repeat. Continue repeating the stroke at finger-width increments down the forehead to the eyebrows.

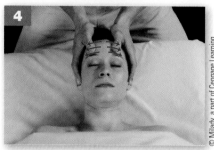

5 Beginning at one side of the forehead, do alternating diagonal gliding strokes or crisscross gliding strokes from the eyebrows into the hairline. Begin with the pads of the fingers of one hand placed at the level of the eyebrow, and glide those fingers in the direction of your corresponding shoulder. As soon as the stroke has progressed enough for the fingers of the other hand to be placed in the same place, do so and glide those fingers in the direction of the corresponding shoulder. Continue alternating diagonal strokes across the forehead and back again.

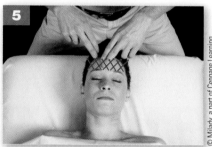

6 Grasp across the bridge of the nose with the thumb and finger and gently traction superiorly and away from the face.

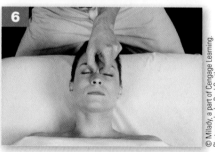

7 Apply light gliding strokes from the nose to the side of the eye socket; first just superior to the supraorbital ridge, then just inferior to the supraorbital ridge, then just inferior to the infraorbital ridge, and finally over the infraorbital ridge. The muscle tissue around the eyes is perhaps the most delicate on the body, so massage movements likewise must be gentle. (*Caution:* Avoid strokes around the eyes if the client is wearing contact lenses.)

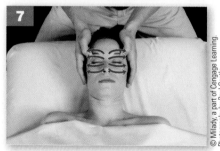

Massage the Face continued

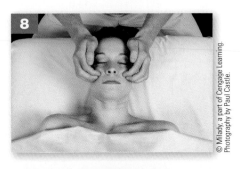

8 Continue to massage with gentle circular friction, using the pads of the fingers, beside the nose from the eyes to the mouth and laterally beneath the zygomatic arch. Gently press upward under the zygomatic arch with the fingertips. The medial portion of the zygomatic arch is the site of the origin of several mimetic muscles (muscles of expression). Although the friction massage is circular, the intention is to massage these muscles of expression in an upward direction.

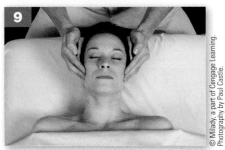

9 Massage the masseter muscle with circular friction and gliding strokes with the thumb or fingers from the lateral aspect of the zygomatic arch to the ramus of the mandible. The parotid salivary gland is located over the posterior aspect of the masseter muscle and the temperomandibular joint (TMJ). Avoid pressure over the parotid gland and the TMJ.

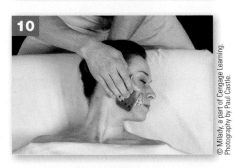

10 Tender points or trigger points are common in the masseter muscle on the mandible. These can be addressed with gentle point compression for 6 to 10 seconds, repeated two or three times followed by gliding movements.

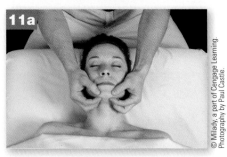

11 Continue to massage along the mandible from the tip of the chin to the ramus of the jaw. The fingers apply gentle circular friction inferior to the mandible while the thumbs gently massage above the ridge. Gently massage under the chin with the pads of the fingers while massaging the area from the lower lip to the chin with the thumbs. Finish with gliding strokes from the chin to the ear.

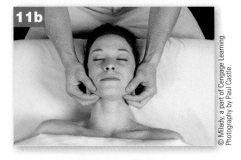

12 Apply light gliding strokes with the fingertips or thumbs from the centerline of the face to the side of the head with an upward orientation in increments starting at the chin, then under and above the lips.

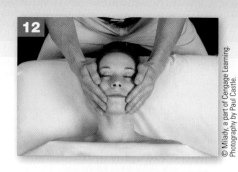

13 Continue digital gliding movements beginning next to the nose and under the eyes and proceeding laterally to the hairline and the temples.

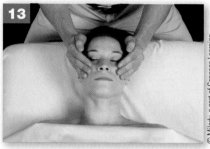

14 Apply gliding movements from the center of the forehead to the temples.

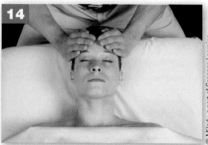

15 Complete the face massage by placing both hands lightly over the entire face, the thenar eminence on the forehead, and fingertips at the outer edge of the lips. Hold still for a moment, allowing the client to sink further into a relaxed state.

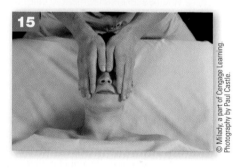

Massage the Face

Rubrics are used in education for organizing and interpreting data gathered from observations of student performance. It is a clearly developed scoring document used to differentiate between levels of development in a specific skill performance or behavior. Rubrics are provided in this supplement for use as either a self-assessment tool to aid the student in behavior development or as an educator assessment tool to determine competence. Space is provided to record steps needed for further growth and improvement.

Performance is evaluated according to the following scale:

1 **Development Opportunity:** There is little or no evidence of competency; Assistance is needed; Performance includes multiple errors.

2 **Fundamental:** There is beginning evidence of competency; Task is completed alone; Performance includes few errors.

3 **Competent:** There is detailed and consistent evidence of competency; Task is completed alone; Performance includes rare errors.

4 **Strength:** There is detailed evidence of highly creative, inventive, mature presence of competency. Space is provided for comments to assist you in improving your performance and achieving a higher rating.

PERFORMANCE ASSESSED	1	2	3	4	IMPROVEMENT PLAN
Procedure					
1. With the client lying face up (supine) on the massage table, properly draped, the practitioner is at the head of the table and has taken a moment to calm their thoughts, center, and ground.					
2. Made initial contact by placing the fingers on the frontal eminence.					
3. After a moment or when a pulse is felt, the fingers were pulled toward the hairline.					
4. Applied gliding strokes with the thumbs from the midline of the forehead to the temples, concluded with circular friction on the temples. Repeated gliding on the forehead with the thumbs in increments from the hairline to the eyebrows.					
5. Applied alternating, diagonal gliding strokes from the eyebrows to the hairline using the fingertips.					
6. Grasped the bridge of the nose between the thumb and index finger and applied a gentle traction away from the face.					
7a. Applied gentle gliding strokes from the nose to the side of the eye socket, just above the supraorbital ridge of the eye.					
7b. Repeated the gliding stroke just inferior to the supraorbital ridge of the eye.					

PERFORMANCE ASSESSED	1	2	3	4	IMPROVEMENT PLAN
7c. Repeated the gliding stroke just inferior to the infraorbital ridge of the eye.					
7d. Repeated the gliding stroke again over the infraorbital ridge of the eye.					
8. Applied gentle circular friction from the nose, over the cheek and under the zygomatic arch.					
9. Continued circular friction down along the masseter muscle. Avoided pressure on the parotid gland.					
10. Located and applied pressure to the trigger points in the masseter muscle.					
11. Applied circular friction along the mandible from the tip of the chin to the ramus of the jaw.					
12. Applied gliding strokes from the centerline of the face to the side of the head, starting at the chin then under and above the lips.					
13. Continued digital gliding movements beginning next to the nose and under the eyes and proceeding laterally to the hairline and the temples.					
14. Applied gliding movements from the center of the forehead to the temples.					
15. Completed the face massage by placing the palms of the hands over the face.					

Massage the Scalp

Overview

To massage the scalp thoroughly, the therapist turns the client's head first one way, then the other, gently and securely supporting the client's head with one hand while massaging with the other.

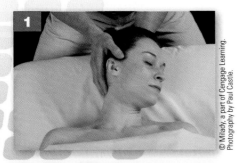

© Milady, a part of Cengage Learning. Photography by Paul Castle.

1 To support the client's head comfortably, the therapist places one hand on either side of the client's head so that the thumbs are positioned just in front of the ears and the fingers extend behind the ears just beyond the occipital ridge. The palms rest comfortably on the cranium so that the hand encircles the ear but does not cover it. Lift the head slightly and turn it on its axis so that it rests comfortably in the cradle of your hand. By using this cranial handle, the therapist should be able to rotate, extend, flex, and even apply gentle traction to the head and neck easily and securely.

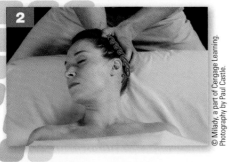

© Milady, a part of Cengage Learning. Photography by Paul Castle.

2 Without lubricant and using the fingertips of the top hand, begin just inferior to the occipital ridge on the side of the head that is exposed and massage the scalp with small circular movements. Use moderate pressure, moving the scalp over the underlying tissues, being careful not to pull the hair. Massage thoroughly across the occipital region and continue the movements across and up the back of the head as you proceed toward the top of the head and above the ear. You may want to turn your hand around to continue the circular friction movements around the ear to cover the entire half of the scalp on the side of the head turned upward.

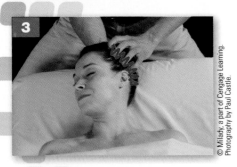

© Milady, a part of Cengage Learning. Photography by Paul Castle.

3 Change the motion of the hand to a quick vibration with the fingers spread apart, starting at the front hairline and progressing toward the occiput, covering the exposed half of the head.

4 Smooth the hair and scalp by combing through the hair with the fingertips from the front hairline to the back.

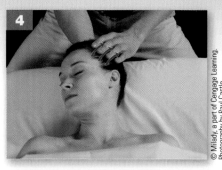

© Milady, a part of Cengage Learning. Photography by Paul Castle.

5 Lay the upper hand on the cranial "handle," turn the head the other way, and do the same procedure on the other side of the scalp. When the second side is completed, return the head to a neutral, forward-facing position.

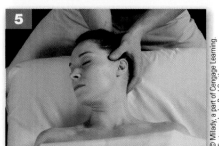

© Milady, a part of Cengage Learning. Photography by Paul Castle.

Massage the Scalp

Rubrics are used in education for organizing and interpreting data gathered from observations of student performance. It is a clearly developed scoring document used to differentiate between levels of development in a specific skill performance or behavior. Rubrics are provided in this supplement for use as either a self-assessment tool to aid the student in behavior development or as an educator assessment tool to determine competence. Space is provided to record steps needed for further growth and improvement.

Performance is evaluated according to the following scale:

1 **Development Opportunity:** There is little or no evidence of competency; Assistance is needed; Performance includes multiple errors.

2 **Fundamental:** There is beginning evidence of competency; Task is completed alone; Performance includes few errors.

3 **Competent:** There is detailed and consistent evidence of competency; Task is completed alone; Performance includes rare errors.

4 **Strength:** There is detailed evidence of highly creative, inventive, mature presence of competency. Space is provided for comments to assist you in improving your performance and achieving a higher rating.

PERFORMANCE ASSESSED	1	2	3	4	IMPROVEMENT PLAN
Preparation					
1. While sitting or standing at the head of the table, held the client's head securely and comfortably with one hand.					
Procedure					
2a. Applied small circular movements to move the scalp over the cranium.					
2b. Used moderate pressure, not pulling the hair; continued the circular movements along the occiput, up the back of the head, and around the ear.					
2c. Turned hand around and continued circular movements around the ear to cover the side of the head that was exposed.					
3. Changed the action of the hand to a quick vibration to massage the scalp from the hairline to the occiput.					
4. Smoothed the hair and scalp by combing through the hair from front to back with the fingertips.					
5. Turned the head the other direction and repeated the same procedure on the other side of the scalp.					

Massage the Ear

Overview

The outer ears extend outward from the ear canal, which penetrates the auricular meatus to the delicate tissues of the inner ear. Because the outer ear is made up of cartilage and an abundance of nerves, it is surprisingly sensitive. For this reason, some clients enjoy having their ears massaged, whereas others are uncomfortable with the practice. French and Chinese therapists have developed auricular therapies with the theory that areas or points of the outer ear are reflexively related to every area and organ in the body. Massaging the points in the ear is thought to have stimulating, relaxing, or rejuvenating effects on areas of the body far removed from the ear. Both ears can be massaged simultaneously.

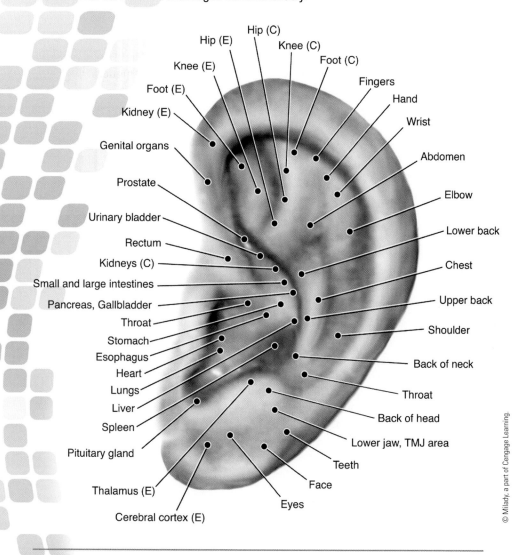

© Milady, a part of Cengage Learning.

Massage the Ear continued

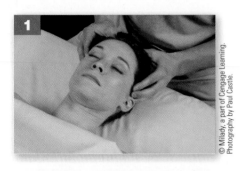

1 Begin by massaging the head all around the ear with circular friction.

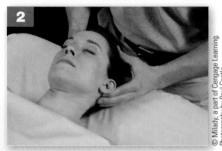

2 Glide around the top and back of the ear where it joins to the head with the edge of your finger (two or three repetitions).

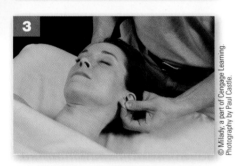

3 Beginning at the lower edge of the ear, using moderate pressure, unroll the outer edge of the ear between your thumb and fingers, applying a slight traction and working all the way around to the upper, anterior aspect of the ear.

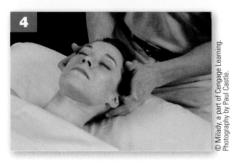

4 Starting at the top front of the ear, use a fingertip (well-trimmed fingernails always) to trace all the valleys and ridges of the ear carefully and with moderate pressure. The thumb can be positioned behind the ear to provide a backing for the manipulation. If any nodules, granular tissue, or other tissue abnormalities are encountered, or if the client says there are tender points, spend a little extra time stimulating these points. These could be an indication of some condition in a related area of the body. You might want to make a note of the tender point for reference to the body area later in the massage or noted in their charts for future treatments.

Part 3: Full Body Relaxation Massage

5 Beginning with the thumbs seated deeply in the center of the ear and the first finger at the base of the ear near the head, grip the ear firmly and slowly pull the ear at an angle away from the head. With digital petrissage, massage the ear between the finger and thumb as you continue tractioning until you reach the outer periphery of the ear. Return the thumb to the center of the ear and repeat the sequence several times, each time in a slightly different direction—inferiorly, inferior-posteriorly, posteriorly, posterior-superiorly, and superiorly.

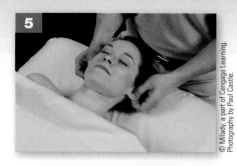

6 Finish by gently tugging inferiorly on the ear lobes, gently grasping and unrolling the outer edges of the ears, and then, using a gliding stroke with the finger, massage the attachment of the ear to the head.

From this point, the massage can continue to the jaw and face or to the neck.

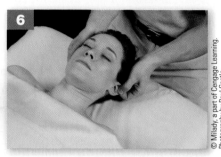

Massage the Ear

Rubrics are used in education for organizing and interpreting data gathered from observations of student performance. It is a clearly developed scoring document used to differentiate between levels of development in a specific skill performance or behavior. Rubrics are provided in this supplement for use as either a self-assessment tool to aid the student in behavior development or as an educator assessment tool to determine competence. Space is provided to record steps needed for further growth and improvement.

Performance is evaluated according to the following scale:

1 **Development Opportunity:** There is little or no evidence of competency; Assistance is needed; Performance includes multiple errors.

2 **Fundamental:** There is beginning evidence of competency; Task is completed alone; Performance includes few errors.

3 **Competent:** There is detailed and consistent evidence of competency; Task is completed alone; Performance includes rare errors.

4 **Strength:** There is detailed evidence of highly creative, inventive, mature presence of competency. Space is provided for comments to assist you in improving your performance and achieving a higher rating.

PERFORMANCE ASSESSED	1	2	3	4	IMPROVEMENT PLAN
Procedure					
1. Applied circular friction to the head and scalp around the ear.					
2. Applied a gliding stroke with the fingers where the ear attaches to the head.					
3a. Started at the lower back of the ear and unrolled the edge between the finger and thumb with a slight traction.					
3b. Continued working around the ear, unrolling the edge, all the way to the upper, anterior aspect of the ear.					
4a. Traced the ridges and valleys of the ear with a well-trimmed and manicured finger.					
4b. Paid attention to any granular tissue or tender points and spent a little extra time stimulating those points.					
5a. Applied digital petrissage and traction with the thumb in the ear and the finger on the back of the ear.					
5b. Repeated the digital petrissage and tractioning of the ear in several directions.					
6a. Gently tugged on the earlobes and gently grasped and unrolled the outer edges of the ears.					
6b. Applied gliding strokes with the sides of the first finger to the attachment of the ear to the head.					

Massage the Neck

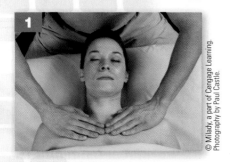

© Milady, a part of Cengage Learning.
Photography by Paul Castle.

1 The practitioner sits or stands at the head of the table to massage the neck. Lubricant is applied to the neck by first putting an adequate amount of lubricant on one hand and then rubbing the hands together. Apply lubricant to the neck with a bilateral-lateral effleurage stroke, beginning at the sternal notch.

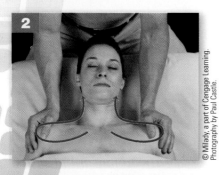

© Milady, a part of Cengage Learning.
Photography by Paul Castle.

2 Leading with the little finger, the effleurage movement proceeds laterally, over the shoulders as the practitioner's hands rotate.

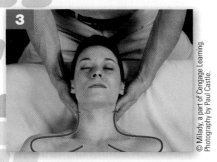

© Milady, a part of Cengage Learning.
Photography by Paul Castle.

3 The bilateral stroke continues up the trapezius and the back of the neck, to the occipital ridge. Repeat the bilateral effleurage stroke three to five times.

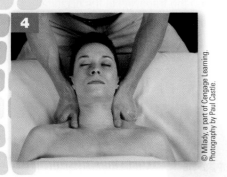

© Milady, a part of Cengage Learning.
Photography by Paul Castle.

4 Apply bilateral petrissage and friction to the neck from the occipital ridge to the shoulders. Begin with circular friction along the occipital ridge then progress down both sides of the neck. Take your time and explore any tight or tender areas.

SERVICE TIP

While massaging the neck, avoid the area of the carotid artery and jugular vein because this can impede circulation to and from the brain and cause the client to become faint.

Massage the Neck continued

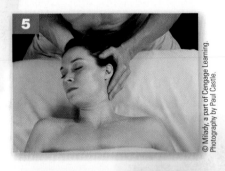

5 Turn the client's head to one side, supporting it with one hand. (Note the hand position for supporting the head with one hand while massaging with the other. The palm of the hand cups the occiput while the thumb and first finger encircle the ear.)

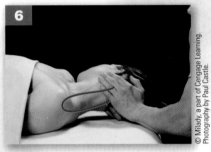

6 Leading with the little finger of the other hand, apply light effleurage strokes, beginning just inferior to (below) the mastoid process (the bony bump below and behind the ear).

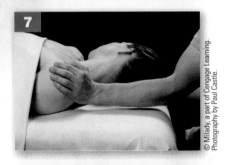

7 Continue the gliding stroke down the lateral aspect of the neck, over the shoulder and around the deltoid muscle.

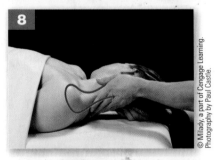

8 The gliding stroke is continuous back up the trapezius to the occipital ridge. Repeat three to five times.

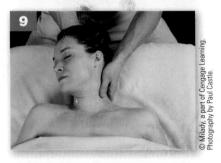

9 Thoroughly knead the same side of the neck, paying attention to any tight areas.

10 Apply circular friction to any congested or tight areas. Begin along the occipital ridge from the midline to the mastoid process. Then proceed down the neck along the levator muscle or the lamina groove to the levator attachment on the scapula.

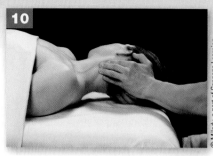

11 Repeat effleurage strokes to that side of the neck and shoulder as in steps 6 to 8.

12 Turn the client's head to the opposite side and repeat the movements as you did in steps 6 to 11.

13 Return the client's head to the central position and repeat bilateral-lateral petrissage and friction to the neck and shoulders. Spend extra time on any areas of tension the fingers palpate.

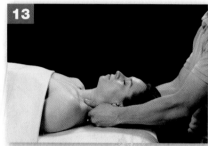

14 Do the following passive joint movements:

14a Tilt the head back with the chin up to extend the neck. Extend the neck by gently lifting segments of the cervical spine toward the ceiling.

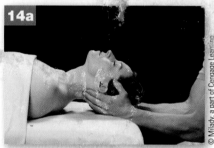

14b Lower the chin to the chest to flex the neck. Gently lift the head and roll the chin toward the chest. (Note the placement of the hands on the occiput.)

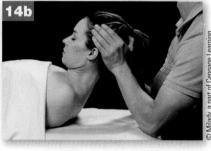

14c Laterally flex the neck, moving the right ear nearer to the right shoulder and gently push the left shoulder toward the feet. Support the head, laterally flexed with one hand and gently push the opposite shoulder toward the feet with the other hand.

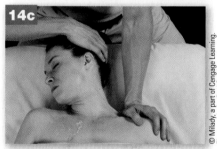

Massage the Neck continued

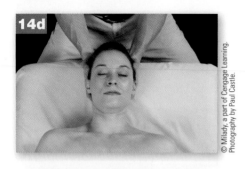

14d Apply a slight traction as the head is returned to a neutral position.

14e Laterally flex the neck, moving the left ear nearer the left shoulder and gently push the right shoulder toward the feet. Then, apply a slight traction while returning the head to a neutral position as shown in step 14d.

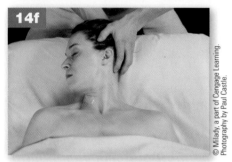

14f Rotate the head to its full range of motion (lateral rotation); first to the right and then to the left. The spine remains elongated and in a straight line.

NOTE: Joint movements of the neck are contraindicated in cases of osteoporosis.

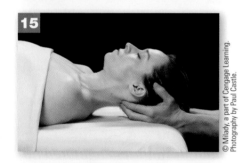

15 Hold the head in the palm of your hand or hook your fingers under the occiput and apply a slight traction to the neck.

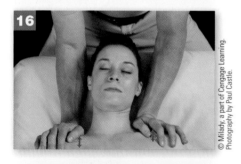

16 Place one hand on each shoulder and alternately push them (gently) toward the feet, providing a gentle rocking motion.

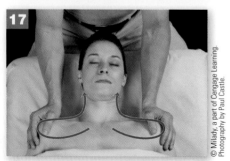

17 Repeat the bilateral-lateral effleurage stroke beginning at the sternal notch and continuing over the shoulders, up the trapezius and the back of the neck, to the occipital ridge three to five times.

Massage the Neck

Rubrics are used in education for organizing and interpreting data gathered from observations of student performance. It is a clearly developed scoring document used to differentiate between levels of development in a specific skill performance or behavior. Rubrics are provided in this supplement for use as either a self-assessment tool to aid the student in behavior development or as an educator assessment tool to determine competence. Space is provided to record steps needed for further growth and improvement.

Performance is evaluated according to the following scale:

1 **Development Opportunity:** There is little or no evidence of competency; Assistance is needed; Performance includes multiple errors.

2 **Fundamental:** There is beginning evidence of competency; Task is completed alone; Performance includes few errors.

3 **Competent:** There is detailed and consistent evidence of competency; Task is completed alone; Performance includes rare errors.

4 **Strength:** There is detailed evidence of highly creative, inventive, mature presence of competency. Space is provided for comments to assist you in improving your performance and achieving a higher rating.

PERFORMANCE ASSESSED	1	2	3	4	IMPROVEMENT PLAN
Procedure					
1. Applied lubricant to the neck with a bilateral-lateral effleurage stroke, beginning at the sternal notch.					
2. Leading with the little finger, the bilateral effleurage stroke proceeded out over and around the shoulder, up along the trapezius and the back of the neck to the occiput.					
3. Repeated bilateral effleurage to the neck three to five times.					
4. Applied bilateral petrissage and friction to the neck from the occiput to the shoulder.					
5. Turned the head to one side, supporting it with one hand.					
6–8. Applied effleurage to the side of the neck and shoulder three to five times.					
9. Applied kneading to the side of the neck and shoulder.					
10. Applied circular friction to the side of the neck, beginning along the occiput and continuing down the neck.					
11. Repeated effleurage to the side of the neck as in step 6 above.					

PERFORMANCE ASSESSED	1	2	3	4	IMPROVEMENT PLAN
12a. Turned the client's head to the other side.					
12b. Applied effleurage to the side of the neck and shoulder three to five times.					
12c. Applied kneading to the side of the neck and shoulder.					
12d. Applied circular friction to the side of the neck, beginning along the occiput and continuing down the neck.					
12e. Repeated effleurage to the side of the neck as in step 6.					
13a. Returned client's head to the neutral position.					
13b. Applied bilateral petrissage to the neck and shoulders.					
13c. Applied bilateral friction to any tight areas of the neck or shoulders.					
14a. Tilted the head back to extend the neck.					
14b. Lowered the chin toward the chest to flex the neck.					
14c. Laterally flexed the neck by moving the right ear nearer to the right shoulder and gently pushing the left shoulder toward the feet.					
14d. Applied a slight traction while returning the head to a neutral position.					
14e. Laterally flexed the neck by moving the left ear nearer the left shoulder and gently pushing the right shoulder toward the feet. Then, applied a slight traction while returning the head to a neutral position.					
14f. Step 1. Rotated the head to the right as far as was comfortable while keeping the spine elongated. Then returned to a neutral position.					
14f. Step 2. Rotated the head to the left as far as was comfortable while keeping the spine elongated. Then returned to a neutral position.					
15. Held the head in the palm of the hands with the fingers hooked under the occipital ridge and applied traction to the neck.					
16. Placed one hand on each shoulder and alternately pushed them (gently) toward the feet, providing a gentle rocking motion.					
17. Repeated a light bilateral effleurage beginning at the sternal notch, over the shoulders, and up the trapezius to the occipital ridge.					

Massage the Arms

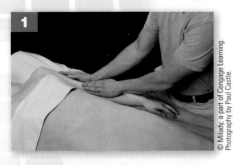

1 Undrape one arm to make contact, and apply lubricant to the client's arm from shoulder to wrist, using light effleurage.

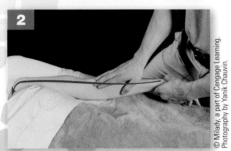

2 Grasp the client's arm at the level of the wrist, and then put the client's arm in slight traction by holding it with the wrist handle. (Holding on to the client's wrist provides a good "handle" for the practitioner to apply traction or move the body without slipping.) Hold the thumb side handle (the client's wrist) with the arm that is closest to the client.

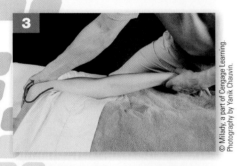

3 Apply effleurage to the lateral aspect of the arm. Begin from the wrist with a gliding stroke up the arm and over the shoulder. Rotate your hand as it travels over the client's shoulder; at the same time, apply slight traction to the handle. Proceed up the back of the neck and then down under the shoulder (trapezius area); glide back to the starting point at the wrist.

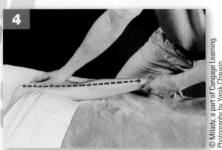

4 The effleurage stroke is continuous with more pressure applied with the effleurage movement distal to proximal (from wrist to neck); lighter pressure is applied proximal to distal with the return stroke. Repeat three to five times.

Massage the Arms continued

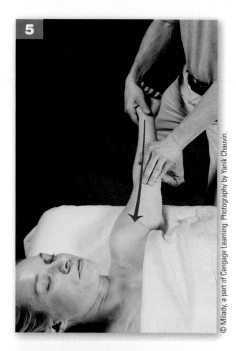

5 Switch the client's wrist handle to your other hand (the outside hand). Apply effleurage with firmer pressure up the medial aspect of the arm.

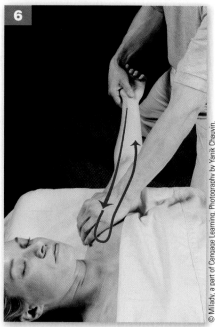

6 Continue the effleurage up and over the shoulder and with slightly lighter pressure back down the arm to about the elbow.

7 Apply effleurage from the elbow back up into the axillary area. Then return to the wrist with lighter pressure. Perform effleurage to the medial aspect of the arm again three to five times.

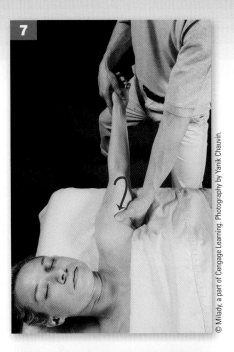

8 Using both hands, grasp the arm at shoulder level and apply petrissage, directing individual movements toward the shoulder while moving proximal to distal down the arm to the client's hand. On the upper arm, use both hands to alternately knead the biceps and triceps.

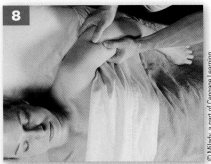

9 Continue to work down the arm while directing each petrissage stroke toward the heart. On the forearm, alternately knead the wrist flexors and extensors.

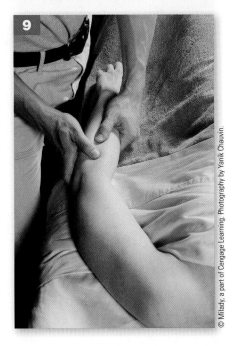

Massage the Arms continued

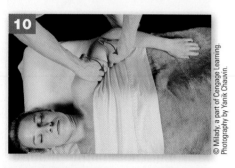

© Milady, a part of Cengage Learning. Photography by Yanik Chauvin.

10 Apply wringing movements from the shoulder to the wrist.

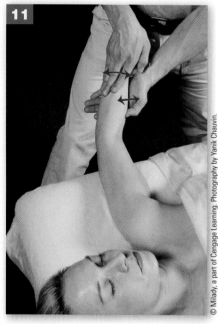

© Milady, a part of Cengage Learning. Photography by Yanik Chauvin.

11 Apply rolling, beginning close to the shoulder and working down the arm to the hand.

12 Apply V-stroke effleurage from wrist to elbow on the medial and lateral sides of the forearm.

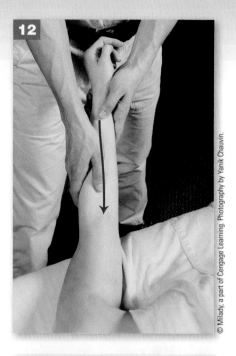

13 Apply fulling to the arm.

14 Repeat effleurage to the medial and lateral side of the arm, as in steps 2 to 7.

15 Massage the hand according to the suggestions in the following procedure entitled *Massage the Hand and Joint Movements for the Hands and Arms*. Proceed to do joint movements on the arm and hand.

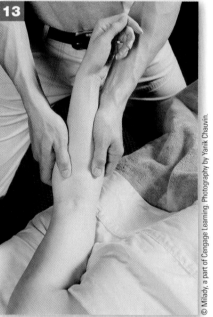

PERFORMANCE RUBRICS

Massage the Arms

Rubrics are used in education for organizing and interpreting data gathered from observations of student performance. It is a clearly developed scoring document used to differentiate between levels of development in a specific skill performance or behavior. Rubrics are provided in this supplement for use as either a self-assessment tool to aid the student in behavior development or as an educator assessment tool to determine competence. Space is provided to record steps needed for further growth and improvement.

Performance is evaluated according to the following scale:

1 **Development Opportunity:** There is little or no evidence of competency; Assistance is needed; Performance includes multiple errors.

2 **Fundamental:** There is beginning evidence of competency; Task is completed alone; Performance includes few errors.

3 **Competent:** There is detailed and consistent evidence of competency; Task is completed alone; Performance includes rare errors.

4 **Strength:** There is detailed evidence of highly creative, inventive, mature presence of competency. Space is provided for comments to assist you in improving your performance and achieving a higher rating.

PERFORMANCE ASSESSED	1	2	3	4	IMPROVEMENT PLAN
Procedure					
1. Undraped one arm in preparation for massage. Applied lubricant from shoulder to wrist with light effleurage.					
2. Grasped the client's wrist with the hand closest to the table, applied slight traction, and applied effleurage with the other hand to the lateral side of the arm.					
3. Continued the effleurage stroke up the lateral aspect of the arm, over the shoulder, up the side of the neck, down the trapezius, to the back of the shoulder, and then returned to the wrist three to five times.					
4. Applied more pressure distal to proximal (from the wrist to the shoulder and neck) and less pressure on the return stroke.					
5-7. Switched the client's wrist handle to the other and applied effleurage to the medial side of the arm three to five times.					
8. Applied two-handed petrissage to the arm from the shoulder to the wrist. On the upper arm, alternately knead the biceps and the triceps.					
9. Continued petrissage on the lower arm, alternately kneading the flexors and extensors.					

PERFORMANCE ASSESSED	1	2	3	4	IMPROVEMENT PLAN
10. Applied wringing to the arm from the shoulder to the wrist.					
11. Applied rolling to the arm from the shoulder to the wrist.					
12. Applied deeper, V-stroke effleurage from the wrist to the elbow on the lateral and medial side of the wrist.					
13. Applied fulling to the forearm.					
14. Repeated effleurage to the medial and lateral sides of the arm three to five times.					

Notes

_____

_____

_____

_____

_____

_____

_____

_____

_____

Massage the Hand and Joint Movements for the Hands and Arms

Overview

Hand massage is a continuation of the arm massage. At the completion of massaging the hand, joint movements of the fingers, hand, wrist, elbow, and shoulder are incorporated.

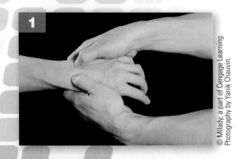

1 Thoroughly knead the back of the hand.

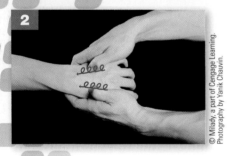

2 Apply circular friction to the back of the hand and wrist.

© Milady, a part of Cengage Learning.
Photography by Yanik Chauvin.

3 Turn the hand over and apply petrissage and friction to the palm of the hand.

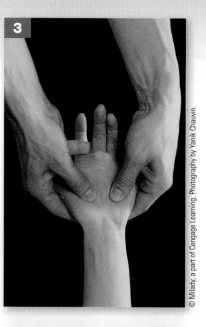

4 With the client's elbow resting on the table, hold the hand upright and massage the palm with your thumbs using circular movements in opposite directions.

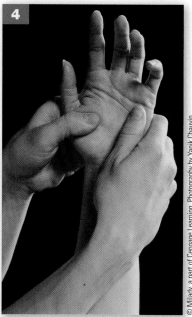

Massage the Hand and Joint Movements for the Hands and Arms continued

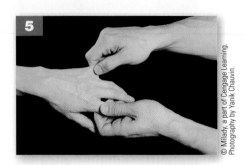

5 Do petrissage on each finger, including a joint movement.

© Milady, a part of Cengage Learning. Photography by Yanik Chauvin.

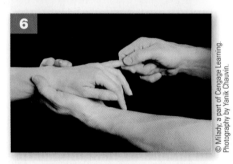

6 Gently squeeze, twist, and circumduct each digit, beginning at the base of each finger and working toward the tip.

© Milady, a part of Cengage Learning. Photography by Yanik Chauvin.

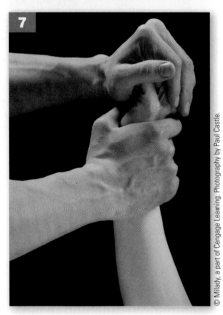

7 Flex the fingers at each phalangial joint.

© Milady, a part of Cengage Learning. Photography by Paul Castle.

8 Extend and circumduct the fingers in unison.

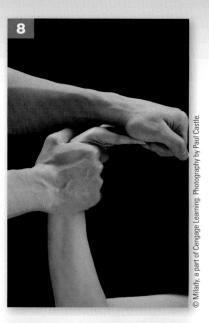

9 Stabilize the elbow on the massage table and flex, extend, and circumduct the wrist. Note the interlacing of the fingers.

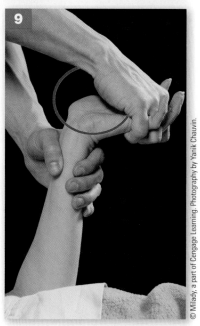

Massage the Hand and Joint Movements for the Hands and Arms continued

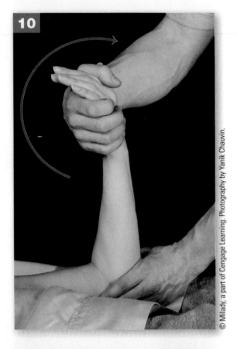

© Milady, a part of Cengage Learning. Photography by Yanik Chauvin.

10 Rotate and circumduct the forearm at the elbow. Note how the elbow is supported by the free hand.

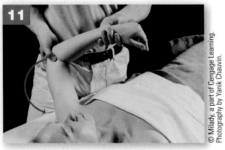

© Milady, a part of Cengage Learning. Photography by Yanik Chauvin.

11 Rotate and circumduct the arm at the shoulder joint by moving the elbow in large circles. Note how the wrist is supported to keep the client's hand from hitting them in the face.

12 Extend the arm above the client's head and apply a slight traction to stretch the entire arm.

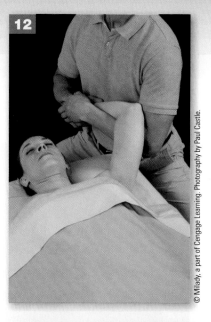

13 While the arm is extended above the head, apply effleurage from the elbow into and past the axillary area.

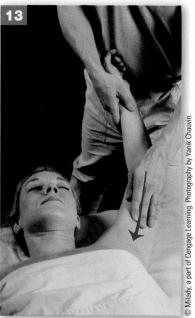

14 Apply traction at the wrist while moving the arm from a position above the client's head and back down to the side.

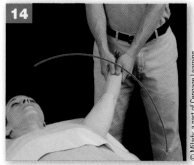

Massage the Hand and Joint Movements for the Hands and Arms continued

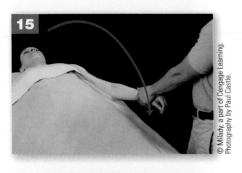

15 Maintain traction on the arm as you move from the head of the table back to the client's side.

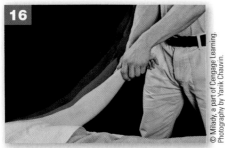

16 Continue a slight traction with a firm, yet gentle grasp of the client's wrist and shake and vibrate the arm up and down.

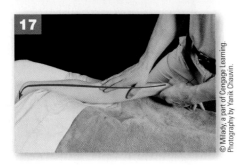

17 Apply a final effleurage to the lateral aspect of the entire length of the arm three to five times.

18 Apply a final effleurage to the medial aspect of the entire length of the arm three to five times.

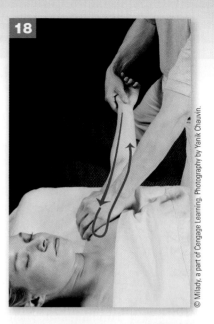

19 Apply superficial feather (nerve) strokes from the neck, down the arm, and to the fingertips.

20 Re-drape the client as necessary, and repeat the arm and hand massage for the other arm and hand.

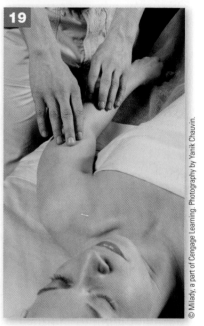

Massage the Hand and Joint Movements for the Hands and Arms

Rubrics are used in education for organizing and interpreting data gathered from observations of student performance. It is a clearly developed scoring document used to differentiate between levels of development in a specific skill performance or behavior. Rubrics are provided in this supplement for use as either a self-assessment tool to aid the student in behavior development or as an educator assessment tool to determine competence. Space is provided to record steps needed for further growth and improvement.

Performance is evaluated according to the following scale:

1 **Development Opportunity:** There is little or no evidence of competency; Assistance is needed; Performance includes multiple errors.

2 **Fundamental:** There is beginning evidence of competency; Task is completed alone; Performance includes few errors.

3 **Competent:** There is detailed and consistent evidence of competency; Task is completed alone; Performance includes rare errors.

4 **Strength:** There is detailed evidence of highly creative, inventive, mature presence of competency. Space is provided for comments to assist you in improving your performance and achieving a higher rating.

PERFORMANCE ASSESSED	1	2	3	4	IMPROVEMENT PLAN
Hand massage is a continuation of the arm massage and will include joint movements of the hand and arm.					
Procedure					
1. Applied kneading to the back of the hand.					
2. Applied circular friction to the back of the hand and wrist.					
3. Turned the hand over and applied friction and petrissage to the palm of the hand.					
4. With the client's elbow supported on the table, held the client's hand upright and massaged the palm with their thumbs using circular movements in opposite directions.					
5. Applied petrissage to each finger.					
6. Gently squeezed, twisted, and circumducted each finger.					
7. Flexed the fingers at each phalangial joint.					
8. Extended and circumducted the fingers in unison.					
9. Flexed, extended, and circumducted the wrist with the elbow supported on the table.					
10. Rotated and circumducted the forearm at the elbow.					

PERFORMANCE ASSESSED	1	2	3	4	IMPROVEMENT PLAN
11. Rotated and circumducted the arm at the shoulder joint.					
12. Extended the client's arm over the head and applied a slight traction to stretch the arm.					
13. Applied effleurage to the extended arm from the elbow down past the axillary area.					
14. Applied traction to the arm while moving it back down to the side of the body.					
15. Maintained traction on the arm as the therapist moved from the head of the table back to the client's side.					
16. Grasped the wrist and applied shaking to the arm.					
17. Applied effleurage to the lateral side of the arm three to five times					
18. Applied effleurage to the medial side of the arm three to five times.					
19. Applied a feather (nerve) stroke from the neck to the fingertips.					
20. Re-draped the arm.					

Notes

_____

_____

_____

_____

_____

_____

_____

Massage the Feet

Overview

Move to the feet, maintaining contact by using a light, brushing stroke down the side of the body. Pause momentarily to allow the client to sense where you are before you begin massaging the feet.

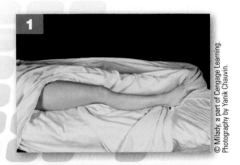

© Milady, a part of Cengage Learning.
Photography by Yanik Chauvin.

1 Undrape one foot and leg to the hip.

2 Use just enough lubricant to allow your hands to work smoothly. (Sometimes no lubricant is needed on the feet.)

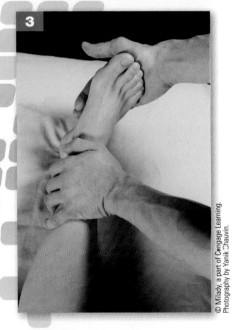

© Milady, a part of Cengage Learning.
Photography by Yanik Chauvin.

3 Apply effleurage to each aspect of the foot. Apply gliding strokes distal to proximal ending just past the ankle on the dorsal, medial, and lateral sides, and plantar surface (bottom) of the foot.

4 Apply petrissage and friction to the plantar surface (bottom) of the foot from the ball of the foot to the heel.

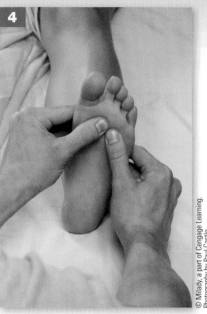

5 Use a closed fist or heel of the hand to do deep gliding to the plantar surface of the foot from the toes to the heel.

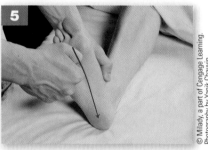

6 Apply kneading movements on the dorsal and plantar surfaces of the foot from the toes up to the ankle.

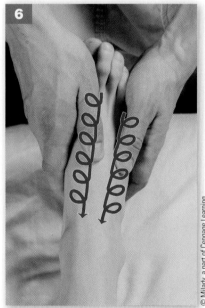

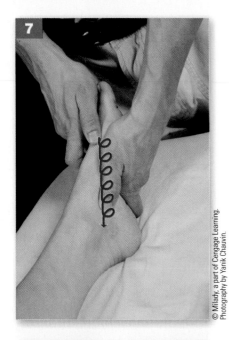

© Milady, a part of Cengage Learning. Photography by Yanik Chauvin.

7 Apply small circular friction movements between each of the tendons on the dorsal, medial, and lateral sides of the foot.

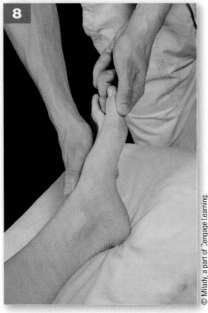

© Milady, a part of Cengage Learning. Photography by Yanik Chauvin.

8 Massage and circumduct each toe, working from the base to the tip of each digit.

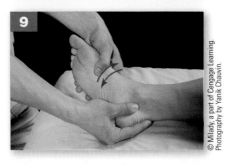

© Milady, a part of Cengage Learning. Photography by Yanik Chauvin.

9 Apply wringing movements to the foot to stretch and rotate the tarsals and metatarsals.

10 Apply dorsal flexion to the toes, and then to the entire foot.

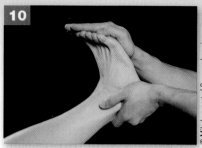

11 Apply plantar flexion to the toes and ankle.

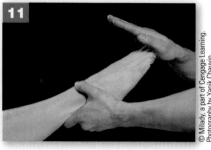

12 Apply a slight stretch to the Achilles tendon.

13 Repeat this entire procedure on the other foot.

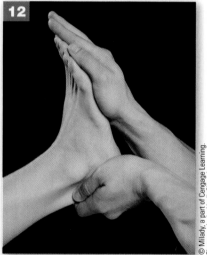

SERVICE TIP

You can choose to work on adjacent parts of the body in sequence (from one part to the adjoining part) rather than interrupting the flow of movement. After working on the foot, proceed directly to the front of the leg. Then continue to the other foot and leg.

Massage the Feet

Rubrics are used in education for organizing and interpreting data gathered from observations of student performance. It is a clearly developed scoring document used to differentiate between levels of development in a specific skill performance or behavior. Rubrics are provided in this supplement for use as either a self-assessment tool to aid the student in behavior development or as an educator assessment tool to determine competence. Space is provided to record steps needed for further growth and improvement.

Performance is evaluated according to the following scale:

1 **Development Opportunity:** There is little or no evidence of competency; Assistance is needed; Performance includes multiple errors.

2 **Fundamental:** There is beginning evidence of competency; Task is completed alone; Performance includes few errors.

3 **Competent:** There is detailed and consistent evidence of competency; Task is completed alone; Performance includes rare errors.

4 **Strength:** There is detailed evidence of highly creative, inventive, mature presence of competency. Space is provided for comments to assist you in improving your performance and achieving a higher rating.

PERFORMANCE ASSESSED	1	2	3	4	IMPROVEMENT PLAN
Procedure					
1. Moved from the arm to the foot, maintaining contact with a light, brushing stroke down the side of the body. Undraped one foot and leg up to the hip.					
2. (Optional) Applied enough lubricant to allow your hands to work smoothly. Sometimes no lubricant is needed on the feet.					
3. Applied effleurage to the foot from the toes to just past the ankle.					
4. Applied petrissage and friction to the plantar surface of the foot.					
5. Used a closed fist or heel of the hand to do deep gliding to the plantar surface of the foot from the toes to the heel.					
6. Applied kneading movements to the dorsal side of the foot.					
7. Applied circular friction movements between the tendons on the dorsal, lateral, and medial sides of the foot.					
8. Applied digital friction and circumduction to each toe.					
9. Applied wringing movements to the foot.					
10. Applied dorsal flexion to the toes and ankle.					
11. Applied plantar flexion to the toes and ankle.					
12. Applied a stretch to the Achilles tendon.					
13. Repeated the entire procedure to the other foot.					

Massage the Front of the Legs

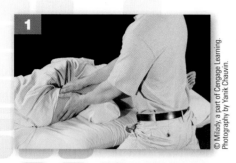

© Milady, a part of Cengage Learning.
Photography by Yanik Chauvin.

1 Apply lubricant with light and continuous effleurage. Warm the lubricant by rubbing it between your two hands and then distributing it along the entire length of the leg with a long, light continuous effleurage stroke. Note: A small bolster can be placed under the knees to reduce tension in the lower back and provide more comfort for the client.

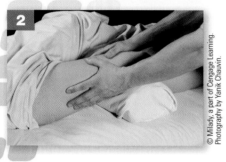

© Milady, a part of Cengage Learning.
Photography by Yanik Chauvin.

2 Apply effleurage with both hands, beginning at the ankle. Apply effleurage to the entire leg by leading with one hand on the lateral side of the leg and the other hand on the medial aspect of the leg. Your hands should span the entire front of the leg. Hand pressure can be increased with each distal to proximal effleurage stroke, returning with light pressure to the starting point. The lateral hand starts at the ankle, continues up the lateral aspect of the anterior leg, all the way to the anterior superior iliac spine (ASIS), along the iliac crest, and glides back to the starting point. Simultaneously the medial hand progresses from the ankle, up the medial aspect of the leg to just below the groin, and turns as it returns lightly along the medial aspect of the leg to the beginning point at the ankle in unison with the lateral hand. Repeat these movements three to five times.

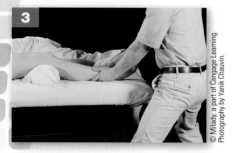

© Milady, a part of Cengage Learning.
Photography by Yanik Chauvin.

3 The leg is the longest part of the body. Be sure to use proper body mechanics and movement when applying long strokes to the leg. Note the body position when beginning the long effleurage stroke.

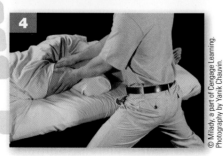

© Milady, a part of Cengage Learning.
Photography by Yanik Chauvin.

4 As the effleurage progress up the leg, shift the body weight to the other foot, maintaining good body alignment.

Massage the Front of the Legs continued

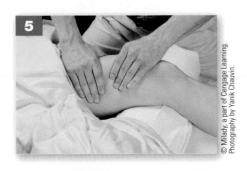

5 Apply petrissage to the thigh. The thigh might require several passes up and down with this stroke because it is a large area.

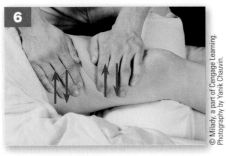

6 Apply wringing to the anterior thigh.

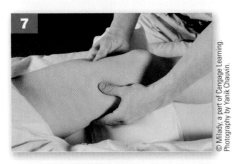

7 Apply fulling to the anterior thigh.

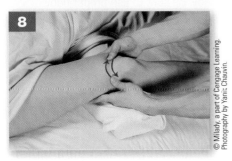

8 Digital petrissage is applied to the more tendinous areas around the patella. Trace circles around the patella in opposite directions with your thumb.

9 Repeat effleurage, as in step 2.

Optional Position: Bending the Knee

Overview

The following is an optional position for leg massage. In this position, the anterior, lateral, and posterior aspects of the calf and thigh can be massaged easily. Position the client's foot flat on the table with the knee bent and the foot 16 to 18 inches (406.4 mm to 457.2 mm) from the buttocks. Wrap the foot with the drape, and brace the leg either with your knee or by sitting on the table near the client's toes to keep the leg from sliding. Be sure the draping is secure to ensure modesty of the pelvic area.

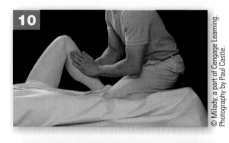

10 With the leg in the bent-knee position, apply effleurage from ankle to knee.

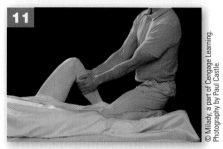

11 Apply petrissage from the ankle to the knee, addressing the tibialis anterior and the gastrocnemius.

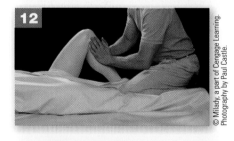

12 Repeat effleurage from ankle to knee.

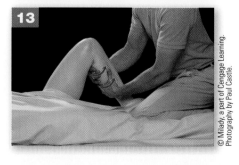

13 While keeping the knee bent, apply a variety of friction techniques from ankle to knee. Pay special attention to areas that seem to be more congested or tight. Apply rolling, wringing, or cross-fiber friction in areas of tension.

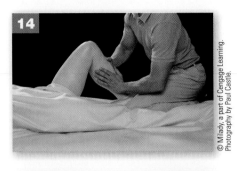

14 Repeat effleurage from ankle to knee.

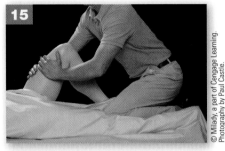

15 Keeping the leg in the bent-knee position, apply effleurage from the knee to the hip around the entire circumference of the thigh.

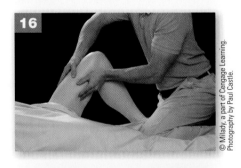

16 Apply petrissage to the entire thigh. Make several passes to cover the entire circumference of the leg.

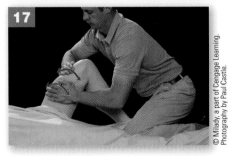

17 Apply wringing to the thigh.

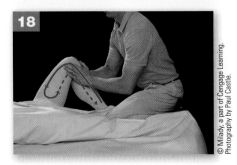

18 Follow with effleurage to the entire leg.

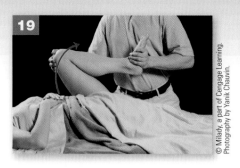

19 Apply joint movements. Grasp the ankle with one hand, and place the other hand near the knee. Flex the knee and the hip and move the knee toward the chest. Pay attention to the degree of flexibility, and move the limbs firmly but not forcefully to their maximum range of movement. It is beneficial to have the client breathe deeply and then exhale as you apply downward pressure on the knee toward the chest.

© Milady, a part of Cengage Learning. Photography by Yanik Chauvin.

SERVICE TIP

During joint movements of the leg it is essential to practice proper draping to ensure the client's modesty and comfort. Secure the draping across the hip and groin area. This is a good time to have the client assist by holding the draping securely while the practitioner performs the joint movements.

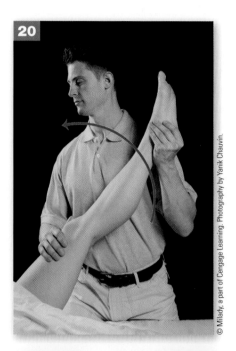

20 Perform hip flexion and stretch the hamstrings by moving your hand around to grasp the ankle at the level of the Achilles tendon; then elevate the foot toward the ceiling to extend the leg. Extend the knee and hip until the leg is straight and then stretch the hamstrings to their maximum range of movement by moving the foot toward the ceiling until a slight stretch is felt.

© Milady, a part of Cengage Learning. Photography by Yanik Chauvin.

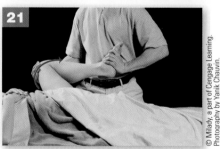

21 Hip rotation is performed by flexing the client's knee, bringing it toward the chest; rotate the bent leg laterally, retaining slight pressure on the knee to maintain full range of motion as the leg rotates outward.

© Milady, a part of Cengage Learning. Photography by Yanik Chauvin.

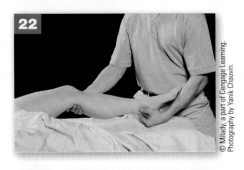

© Milady, a part of Cengage Learning.
Photography by Yanik Chauvin.

22 Return the leg to the table by continuing the hip rotation and slowly straightening the leg. Your hand should support the back of the leg to prevent hyperextension as the leg is returned to the table. Repeat step 21 and 22 twice.

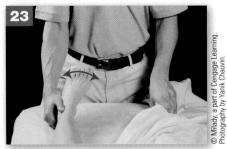

© Milady, a part of Cengage Learning.
Photography by Yanik Chauvin.

23 Move to the foot of the table and grasp the heel (handle) with the lateral hand (the one toward the outside of the leg you were working on). Rotate the foot and leg in the hip socket. This movement is back and forth, and the foot movement resembles that of a windshield wiper.

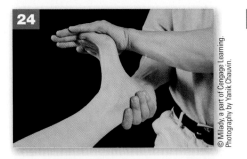

© Milady, a part of Cengage Learning.
Photography by Yanik Chauvin.

24 Dorsal flex the foot and ankle.

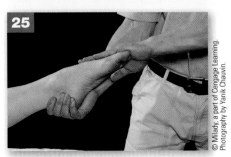

© Milady, a part of Cengage Learning.
Photography by Yanik Chauvin.

25 Plantar flex the foot and ankle.

26 Apply traction to the leg by grasping the heel with one hand and placing the other hand over the client's instep to apply slight traction. Maintaining the same hand positions, shake the leg up and down, bouncing the heel on the table to avoid hyperextension of the knee.

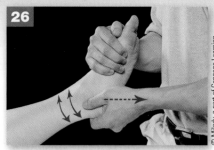

© Milady, a part of Cengage Learning.
Photography by Yanik Chauvin.

27 Apply effleurage to the entire leg three to five times.

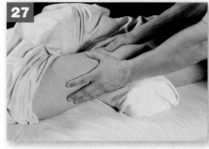

© Milady, a part of Cengage Learning.
Photography by Yanik Chauvin.

28 Apply feather (nerve) strokes from hip to toes, three to five times.

29 Re-drape the leg and proceed to the other foot.

30 Repeat the entire procedure on the other leg.

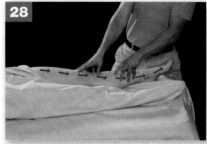

© Milady, a part of Cengage Learning.
Photography by Paul Castle.

Massage the Front of the Legs

Rubrics are used in education for organizing and interpreting data gathered from observations of student performance. It is a clearly developed scoring document used to differentiate between levels of development in a specific skill performance or behavior. Rubrics are provided in this supplement for use as either a self-assessment tool to aid the student in behavior development or as an educator assessment tool to determine competence. Space is provided to record steps needed for further growth and improvement.

Performance is evaluated according to the following scale:

1 **Development Opportunity:** There is little or no evidence of competency; Assistance is needed; Performance includes multiple errors.

2 **Fundamental:** There is beginning evidence of competency; Task is completed alone; Performance includes few errors.

3 **Competent:** There is detailed and consistent evidence of competency; Task is completed alone; Performance includes rare errors.

4 **Strength:** There is detailed evidence of highly creative, inventive, mature presence of competency. Space is provided for comments to assist you in improving your performance and achieving a higher rating.

PERFORMANCE ASSESSED	1	2	3	4	IMPROVEMENT PLAN
Preparation					
The leg is already undraped after the foot massage.					
Procedure					
1. Applied lubricant with a light continuous effleurage stroke.					
2. Applied effleurage to the leg from ankle to hip, leading with the lateral hand, three to five times.					
3-4. Employed good body mechanics while massaging entire length of the leg.					
5. Applied petrissage to the anterior thigh.					
6. Applied wringing to the anterior thigh.					
7. Applied fulling to the anterior thigh.					
8. Applied digital petrissage around the patella.					
9. Repeated effleurage to the entire leg three to five times.					
Optional Position—Bending the Knee					
10. Placed the leg in a bent-knee position. Wrapped the drape over the foot and secured the foot with the practitioner's knee. Applied effleurage from the ankle to the knee.					
11. Applied petrissage from the ankle to the knee.					

PERFORMANCE ASSESSED	1	2	3	4	IMPROVEMENT PLAN
12. Repeated effleurage from the ankle to the knee.					
13a. Applied rolling from the ankle to the knee.					
13b. Applied wringing from the ankle to the knee.					
13c. Applied deeper, cross-fiber friction to areas of tension.					
14. Repeated effleurage from the ankle to the knee.					
15. With the leg in the same, bent-knee position, applied effleurage from the knee to the hip on all aspects of the thigh.					
16. Applied petrissage to the entire thigh.					
17. Applied wringing to the thigh.					
18. Applied effleurage to the entire leg in the bent-knee position three to five times.					
19. Flexed the knee and hip and moved the knee close to the chest.					
20. Extended the leg by elevating the foot toward the ceiling stretching the hamstrings.					
21. Performed hip rotations by flexing the client's knee, bringing it toward the chest; then rotated the bent leg laterally, retaining slight pressure on the knee.					
22. Returned the leg to the table by continuing the hip rotation and slowly straightened the leg. Repeat this procedure twice.					
23. Performed a "windshield wiper" movement with the foot to rotate the femur at the hip.					
24. Dorsal flexed the foot and ankle.					
25. Plantar flexed the foot and ankle.					
26. Applied traction to the leg at the foot and shook the leg up and down.					
27. Applied effleurage to the entire leg three to five times.					
28. Applied feather (nerve) strokes to the leg from the hip to the toes.					
29. Re-draped the leg.					
30. Repeated the entire procedure on the other leg.					

Massaging the Abdomen and Chest

Overview

This part of the massage requires some special considerations. Some clients prefer not to have the abdomen and chest massaged. Always ask before proceeding. The need for draping varies when working with male and female clients. Breast draping is always used on female clients. In some states, breast draping is a legal requirement. Professional standards recommend that proper draping procedures be followed.

The following massage description refers to techniques used on the fully exposed torso, with added comments when using breast draping.

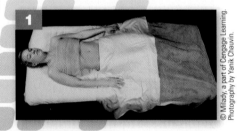

1 In preparation for massage of the abdominal region, use a bolster or pillow to elevate the client's knees and support them so that the abdominal muscles remain relaxed. Draping should be open enough to allow massaging down to one and one-half inch below the navel, and secure enough to avoid exposure of the genital area. Proper draping for abdominal massage includes breast draping for women.

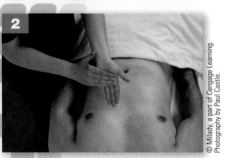

2 To begin, stand to the client's left to apply massage lubricant to the abdomen, chest, and sides of the body. Begin by depositing an adequate amount of lubricant in the palm of your hand; rubbing your hands together; and then distributing the lubricant over the abdomen, chest, and sides of the client.

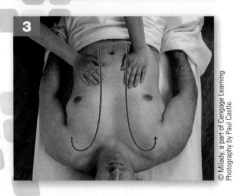

3 On a male client, effleurage strokes on the torso begin at the midline of the abdomen and travels up the chest and out to the shoulders.

On a female client, apply effleurage up the abdomen to just below the breast, out to the sides of the body, and down to the iliac crest. Repeat three to five times.

4 The stroke continues over the shoulders, around and down the axillary areas, and then down the sides of the crest of the ilium.

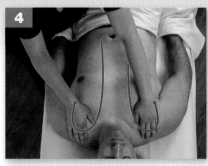

5 Massage back to the center with a turn of your wrist and repeat the movements. When using breast draping, this stroke glides up as far as the drape allows and then laterally over the ribs and down to the iliac crest. Massage should not be done directly over the sensitive area of the nipples on men or women.

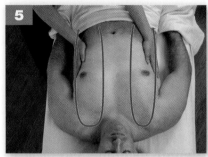

6 Do circular effleurage on the abdomen in a clockwise direction, following the path of the colon. On this stroke, one hand remains in constant contact doing circular massage. The other describes a semicircle beginning at the lower right of the client's abdomen, moving up the right side to the rib cage, across the abdomen just below the rib cage, then down the left side to an area just medial to the hip bone. Abdominal massage should always encourage the natural flow of the large intestines. Repeat the abdominal massage movements several times.

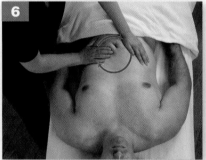

7 Knead the entire abdomen, massaging not only the abdominal muscles but also stimulating the action of the abdominal organs.

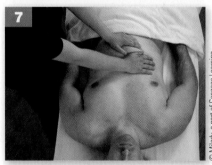

8 To massage the large intestine more thoroughly, apply circular friction to its entire length. Begin in the area of the lower-left quadrant of the abdomen. The circles should be on an oblique (deviation to the vertical or horizontal line) plane of the surface of the abdomen so that pressure is increased and decreased repeatedly over an area about 2 inches square, and at the rate of about 100 circles per minute. This movement encourages the contents of the colon toward the rectum. Proceed slowly back along the course of the colon all the way to the cecum, the first portion of the colon.

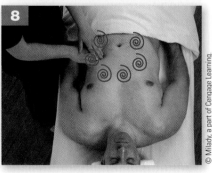

Massaging the Abdomen and Chest continued

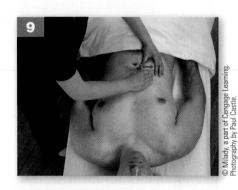

9 Grasp as much of the abdominal tissue as possible and gently lift and shake it.

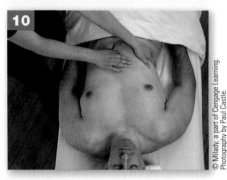

10 Do alternate hand gliding strokes or shingles. Stand to one side of the client and reach over to the opposite side. Alternately pull your hands over the client's body toward you. As one hand nears completion of the stroke, the other begins a stroke. This movement begins just below the crest of the ilium (hip bone) and can continue all the way over the shoulder and up the neck. When working with breast draping, it is necessary to adjust the drape to continue this movement up to the ribs and back down to the hip.

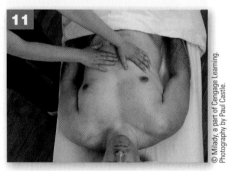

11 When performing shingles, alternate hand gliding the area of the ribs, flex your fingers slightly, and rake gently between the ribs with your fingertips.

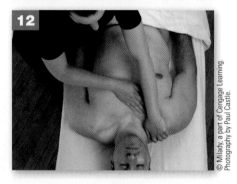

12 Continue to repeat alternate hand gliding strokes (shingles) over the shoulder and up the side of the neck.

13 Apply a deep gliding stroke or a fan stroke from the midline of the abdomen to the side of the body. Begin just inferior to the rib cage and repeat several strokes, moving down the abdomen to the ilium.

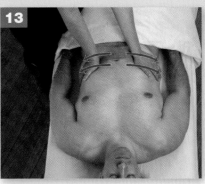

14 Reach under both sides of the lower torso so the fingers are near the lumbar spine. Apply a deep gliding stroke, gently lifting the body slightly off of the table. Continue the stroke around the side of the abdomen toward the midline. Repeat the stroke three to five times.

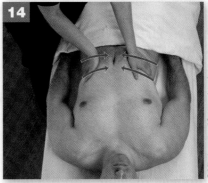

15 Move to the head of the table for the following stroke. This is referred to as the *caring stroke* and is a complete gliding stroke for the torso. This stroke can only be done when breast draping is not used. Begin by placing your fingers (pointing toward each other) with palms flat on the client's skin at the uppermost aspect of the chest.

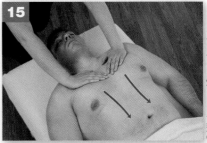

16 Stroke downward over the chest and abdomen to the pubic bone.

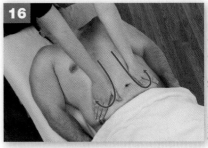

17 Rotate your hands over the client's ilium, around the sides, and back up to the axillary area.

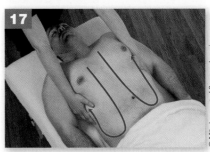

Massaging the Abdomen and Chest continued

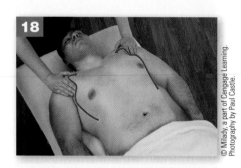

18 Rotate your hands as you continue upward and around the shoulders.

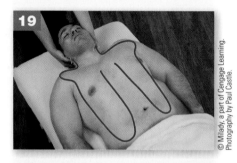

19 Continue the caring stroke up the trapezius muscles to the back of the neck, ending at the occiput.

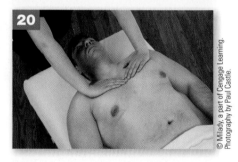

20 Rotate your hands as you move them back down to the starting point. Repeat the movement several times. Beware of any residual tension that your hands might perceive, and spend a few extra moments to work on those areas. Then repeat the caring stroke.

21 This completes the massage of the front of the body. At this point, reposition the top cover or wrap to cover the client, secure the cover, and ask the client to turn over to a prone (face-down) position.

Changing Position

Overview

When it is time for the client to turn over to a prone, face-down position, maintain proper draping to prevent exposure while turning the client. If using a face rest, put it in place at the head of the table.

22 With the client supine, straighten the top cover and hold it in place in three places by leaning against the table with the thighs, and reaching across the client to grasp the top cover at the level of the client's shoulder with one hand and his to mid-thigh with the other.

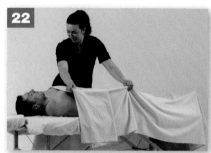

23 Allow some slack in the top cover. Instruct the client to roll over by first facing you and then over on their stomach.

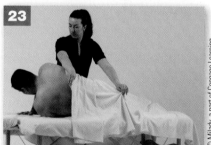

24 Instruct the client to move up on the table until their face is aligned in the face rest. If necessary, adjust the face cradle for comfort. Re-adjust the top cover. Make the client comfortable by supplying a bolster under the ankles, and other supports for the chest or abdomen as needed.

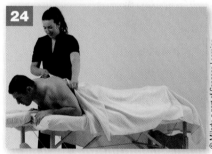

PERFORMANCE RUBRICS

Massaging the Abdomen and Chest

Rubrics are used in education for organizing and interpreting data gathered from observations of student performance. It is a clearly developed scoring document used to differentiate between levels of development in a specific skill performance or behavior. Rubrics are provided in this supplement for use as either a self-assessment tool to aid the student in behavior development or as an educator assessment tool to determine competence. Space is provided to record steps needed for further growth and improvement.

Performance is evaluated according to the following scale:

1 **Development Opportunity:** There is little or no evidence of competency; Assistance is needed; Performance includes multiple errors.

2 **Fundamental:** There is beginning evidence of competency; Task is completed alone; Performance includes few errors.

3 **Competent:** There is detailed and consistent evidence of competency; Task is completed alone; Performance includes rare errors.

4 **Strength:** There is detailed evidence of highly creative, inventive, mature presence of competency. Space is provided for comments to assist you in improving your performance and achieving a higher rating.

PERFORMANCE ASSESSED	1	2	3	4	IMPROVEMENT PLAN
Preparation					
1. In preparation for abdominal massage, a bolster or pillow was placed under the knees to relax the abdominal muscles. Undraped the abdomen of a male client. OR provided proper breast draping and undraped the abdomen of a female client.					
2. Applied lubricant to the abdomen, chest, and sides of the torso.					
3. On a male client, applied effleurage to the entire anterior aspect of the torso; beginning at the middle of the abdomen, up over the chest, and out toward the shoulders.					
4. The stroke continues out around, down the axillary areas, and down the sides to the iliac crest. Repeated three to five times.					
5. On a female client, using breast draping, applied effleurage up the abdomen to just below the breast, out to the sides of the body and down to the iliac crest. Repeated three to five times.					
6. Applied circular effleurage to the abdomen, following the path of the colon.					
7. Applied kneading to the abdomen.					
8. Applied deep circular friction to the colon beginning in the lower-left quadrant of the abdomen and working back along the course of the colon.					

PERFORMANCE ASSESSED	1	2	3	4	IMPROVEMENT PLAN
9. Grasped the skin and superficial tissues over the abdomen, and gently lifted and shook the abdominal area.					
10. Applied deep, alternate hand gliding strokes (shingles) to the far side of the client, beginning at the iliac crest and working up to the ribs and then back down to the iliac crest.					
11. When shingles are applied over the rib area, the tips of the fingers are flexed slightly to rake between the ribs.					
12. Continued alternate hand gliding strokes (shingles) over the shoulder and up the neck.					
13. Applied deep gliding strokes from the midline to the sides of the body from the ribs to the ilium three to five times.					
14. Reached under both sides of the abdomen and applied deep gliding movements from the sides of the body towards the midline three to five times.					
15-20. Moved to the head of the table and applied the caring stroke three to five times.					
21. Re-draped the torso and prepared the client to roll over into a prone position.					
Changing Position					
22. Held the top sheet by leaning against the table with the thighs and holding the top sheet at the level of the client's shoulder and mid-thigh.					
23. Instructed the client to roll over by first facing you and then onto their stomach.					
24. Instructed the client to move up on the table until their face aligns with the face rest. Re-adjusted the top cover.					

Massage the Back of the Legs

1 Undrape the back of one leg. This massage is similar to the procedures for the front of the legs.

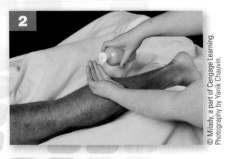

© Milady, a part of Cengage Learning. Photography by Yanik Chauvin.

2 Make contact with the client's skin and apply the massage lubricant with light effleurage strokes. First, apply lubricant to your own hand. Rub your hands together to warm the lubricant and then spread it over the entire area of the leg to be massaged with a light effleurage stroke.

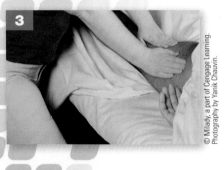

© Milady, a part of Cengage Learning. Photography by Yanik Chauvin.

3 Apply effleurage to the posterior leg, leading with your lateral hand (medial hand following). This stroke begins at the ankles and glides up the leg to the iliac crest and then back to the starting point at the ankles. The lateral hand glides up the lateral aspect of the leg, over the thigh and gluteal muscles, to the iliac crest. The hand rotates and returns to the starting point. Simultaneously, the medial hand glides up the medial/posterior aspect of the leg to about the gluteal crease and then rotates and returns to the starting point at the ankles. Increase the pressure on the upward stroke with each pass. Maintain contact with much lighter pressure on the return stroke. Repeat three to five times.

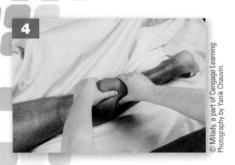

© Milady, a part of Cengage Learning. Photography by Yanik Chauvin.

4 Apply petrissage to the posterior leg, beginning on the calf muscles.

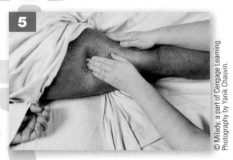

© Milady, a part of Cengage Learning. Photography by Yanik Chauvin.

5 Continue petrissage to include the thigh, upward over the gluteal muscles to the crest of the ilium.

6 Apply fulling to the posterior thigh and calf.

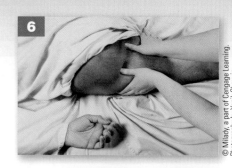

7 Apply wringing to the posterior calf and thigh.

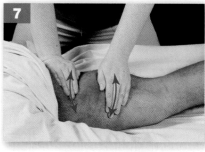

8 Compression movements to the lower leg to enhance local fluid movement.

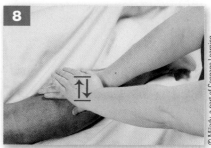

9 Continue compression to the posterior thigh. Avoid heavy movements to the back of the knee.

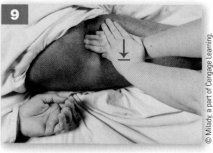

10 Apply deeper friction using braced fingers or the heel of the hand.

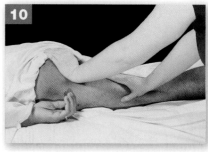

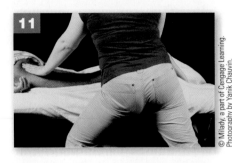

11 When applying deeper movements, always be aware of proper body mechanics.

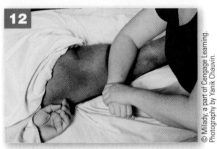

12 Using the forearm can be quite effective for deeper gliding strokes over the hamstrings and the gluteal muscles.

13 Repeat effleurage, as in step 3.

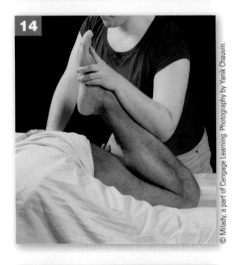

14 Apply joint movements. Grasp the client's ankle and move the foot toward the buttocks with gentle pressure to flex the knee and to stretch the muscles on the front of the thigh.

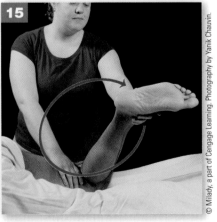

15 Continue by making increasingly larger circles with the ankle to rotate the hip joint. Return the foot to the table.

16 Apply hacking (optional) over the posterior leg. Align the ulnar side of the hand to the orientation of the muscle fibers.

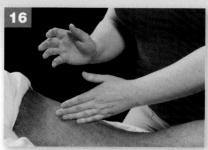

17 Beating percussion applied with a soft fist can be applied to the thicker muscles of the thigh and gluteal area.

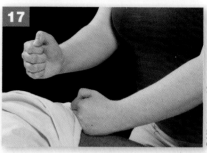

18 Repeat effleurage as a finishing stroke, gently changing to feather (nerve) strokes.

19 Re-drape the leg and repeat the entire procedure on the client's other leg.

Massage the Back of the Legs

Rubrics are used in education for organizing and interpreting data gathered from observations of student performance. It is a clearly developed scoring document used to differentiate between levels of development in a specific skill performance or behavior. Rubrics are provided in this supplement for use as either a self-assessment tool to aid the student in behavior development or as an educator assessment tool to determine competence. Space is provided to record steps needed for further growth and improvement.

Performance is evaluated according to the following scale:

1 **Development Opportunity:** There is little or no evidence of competency; Assistance is needed; Performance includes multiple errors.

2 **Fundamental:** There is beginning evidence of competency; Task is completed alone; Performance includes few errors.

3 **Competent:** There is detailed and consistent evidence of competency; Task is completed alone; Performance includes rare errors.

4 **Strength:** There is detailed evidence of highly creative, inventive, mature presence of competency. Space is provided for comments to assist you in improving your performance and achieving a higher rating.

PERFORMANCE ASSESSED	1	2	3	4	IMPROVEMENT PLAN
Procedure					
1. Undraped the posterior leg.					
2. Applied lubricant to the posterior leg with a thigh effleurage stroke.					
3. Applied effleurage to the posterior leg three to five times.					
4. Applied petrissage to the posterior leg, beginning on the calf.					
5. Applied petrissage to the posterior thigh and gluteal area.					
6. Applied fulling to the posterior thigh and calf.					
7. Applied wringing to the posterior calf and thigh.					
8. Applied compression to the posterior lower leg.					
9. Applied compression to the posterior thigh, avoiding heavy movements to the back of the knee.					
10-11. Applied deeper friction movements with braced fingers being aware of good body mechanics.					
12. Applied deeper gliding movements with the forearm over the posterior thigh and gluteal muscles.					
13. Repeated effleurage to the entire posterior leg three to five times.					

PERFORMANCE ASSESSED	1	2	3	4	IMPROVEMENT PLAN
14. Applied joint movements. Flexed the knee and moved the foot near the gluteal muscles to stretch the anterior thigh muscles.					
15. Circumducted the lower leg at the knee joint to also rotate the femur in the hip socket.					
16. Applied hacking to the posterior leg, aligning the ulnar side of the hand with the orientation of the underlying muscle fibers.					
17. Applied beating percussion to the thicker muscles of the thigh and gluteal area.					
18a. Applied effleurage to the posterior leg three to five times.					
18b. Applied a feather stroke (nerve stroke) to the posterior leg.					
19. Re-draped the posterior leg. Repeated the whole procedure to the other leg.					

Notes

_____

_____

_____

_____

_____

_____

_____

Massage the Back

Overview

No massage is complete without a good back massage. It is important to give a good back massage because the client usually expects and looks forward to this part of the massage. Be sure to pace the massage so that you have ample time to devote to the back massage. Hundreds of manipulations can be performed on the back. They range from extremely superficial stroking to deep tissue work, using elbows and forearms when relieving tension around the spine, pelvis, and shoulders. The following is a basic soothing routine that is guaranteed to leave the recipient in a calm, relaxed state.

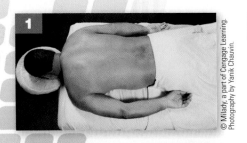

1 Follow proper draping procedures described in Part 1. Fold down the top cover to a level just above the gluteal cleft to expose the back.

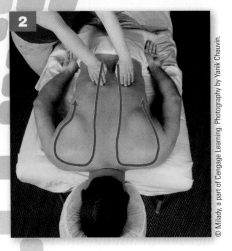

2 Stand to the side of the client. Apply massage lubricant, first to your hands and then to the entire back using long, continuous effleurage strokes.

3 Beginning at the posterior iliac crest, apply long effleurage strokes. Apply long gliding strokes up along the muscles on the sides of the spine to the nape of the neck. Move your hands out and over the shoulders and down the sides of the torso and back down to the hips. Rotate your hands and return to the starting point. Repeat the gliding movement three to five times. Use equal pressure on the pulling and pushing strokes.

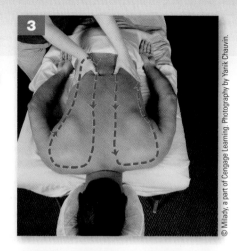

4 Apply petrissage. Begin with the gluteal region on the opposite side of the client from where you are standing. Knead the side of the body from below the ilium up into the axillary area.

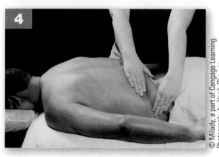

5 Continue over the shoulder to include the trapezius and neck. Move hands medially to a position nearer to the spine (midway between the spine and extreme side of the body), and then knead back down to the gluteal area. Work back up the back along the side of the spine to include the sacrospinalis and erector spinea muscles.

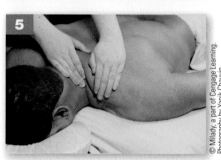

6 Begin at the neck with alternate-hand gliding strokes (shingles) from the side of the body to the spinal process. Move down over the shoulder and down the side to the top of the thigh and then back up to the top of the shoulder.

7 Move to the other side of the table and repeat steps 2 to 6.

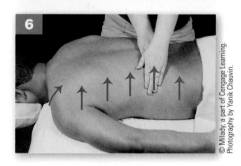

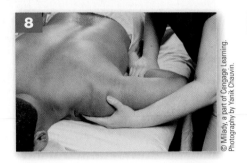

8 Flex the client's elbow (closest to you), and place the client's hand on the table about six inches from the armpit to elevate the medial border of the scapula. Some practitioners prefer to place the client's hand in the small of the back to abduct and elevate the scapula.

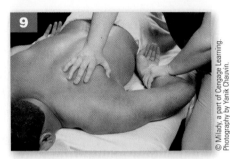

9 In this position, several kneading and friction movements can easily be performed on all sides of the scapula. Special attention should be given to the teres major and minor, trapezius, the rhomboids, and the infraspinatus muscles.

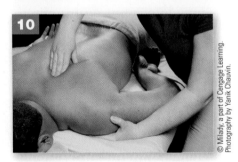

10 Elevate the scapula by lifting the shoulder and applying deep pressure and friction along the vertebral border of the scapula.

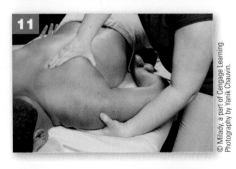

11 Apply joint movement to the shoulder. With the client's hand still in position at the side, grasp the top of the shoulder with one hand. Place your hand under the glenohumeral joint, and use this hold as a handle. Place the other hand just inferior to the scapula so that the inferior angle of the scapula fits neatly into the V formed between your thumb and index finger. Lift and rotate the scapula away from the rib cage. Although this might seem unnecessary, it is very effective in relieving several stress-related shoulder problems. Rotate the shoulder several times in both directions.

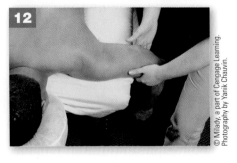

12 Abduct the elbow so that the upper arm is at a square angle from the body and the forearm is relaxed at an angle from the upper arm. Support the arm with both of your hands just proximal to the elbow, allowing the hand and forearm to hang down, and gently swing the hand up and down, allowing the shoulder to rotate in a relaxed manner. Replace the hand and arm to the side of the body.

13 Repeat all the movements, steps 8 to 10, on the other side of the back.

14 Repeat effleurage on the entire back area three to five times.

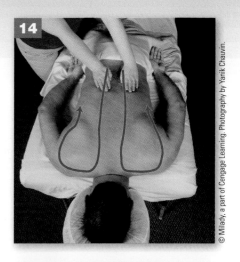

15 Apply a fan stroke, beginning on the upper back and continuing with consecutive gliding strokes from the midline to the sides of the back.

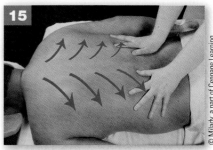

16 Apply wringing friction to the back, moving back and forth across and working all the way up the neck and back down.

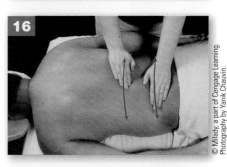

17 Apply circular friction on each side of the spine on the erector spine muscles.

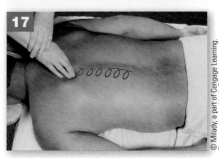

Massage the Back continued

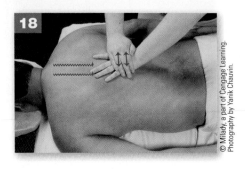

18 Do sacrospinalis vibration. Place the first two fingers of one hand to either side of the client's spine, about 2 inches (50.8 mm) apart. Bend your fingers slightly so that they apply deep pressure on the medial edge of the sacrospinalis muscle and along each side of the spinus process.

Place your other hand on the top of the hand resting on the client's back, and press down firmly while vibrating slowly (about 120 vibrations per minute) from side to side along the client's body. Slowly glide both hands down along the spine, vibrating (jiggling) each portion of the sacrospinalis muscle back and forth about 3 to 10 times. Pay attention to any area that seems especially tense, because these areas should be given extra attention. Work all the way down the spine to the sacrum in this manner. This technique can also be done from the sacrum to the 7th cervical vertebra.

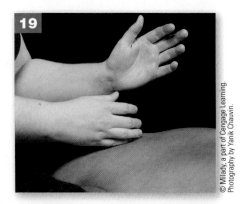

19 At this time, several percussion movements are optional. Hacking can be done lightly over the entire back. (Avoid percussion over the area of the kidneys, the popliteal fossa, or any bony areas.)

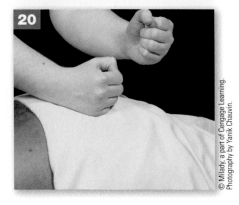

20 Beating movements can be applied over the more muscular areas of the body, including the gluteals and the backs of the legs.

21 Cupping can be done over the lung area to help break up congestion.

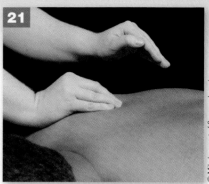

22 To end a stimulating massage, light slapping can be applied over the entire body.

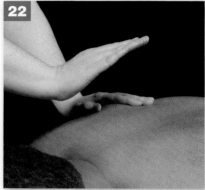

23 A caring stroke completes the back massage. Remember that a caring stroke is an all-inclusive gliding stroke that is applied by standing at the head of the massage table. From a position at the head of the table, place your hands on the upper back so that your fingers nearly touch in the area of the first and second thoracic vertebrae. Apply gliding strokes down the entire length of the spine.

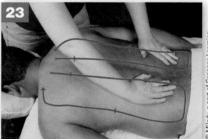

24 Your hands glide over the gluteals and return up the lateral portion of the torso to the axillary area, slide smoothly over the deltoids up the trapezius to the occiput, and return to the starting point. Repeat the movements several times.

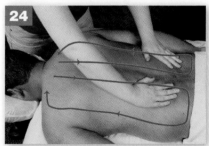

Massage the Back continued

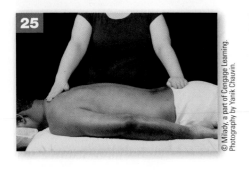

© Milady, a part of Cengage Learning. Photography by Yanik Chauvin.

25 To complete the massage of the entire body, lightly place one hand on the sacrum and the other at the base of the neck and hold the position for several seconds. An option here is to apply a slight rocking motion.

26 Follow the Post-Service procedure described in Part 2. A few reminders are included below:

- Allow the client to relax quietly without being disturbed for several minutes.
- Assist the client to a sitting position. Be sure that draping is properly secured. When the client is reoriented, help the client off of the table if needed and direct them to the dressing area.
- After the client is dressed, take time to answer any questions, make recommendations, collect your fees, and set up the next appointment.
- Following the massage, allow the client to rest for a short while before going out to face the world again. This rest period is beneficial especially if you have done bodywork to the extent that some changes have taken place in the client's physical structure. A few moments of relaxation helps to integrate these changes into the client's psychological and neurologic senses.

Massage the Back

Rubrics are used in education for organizing and interpreting data gathered from observations of student performance. It is a clearly developed scoring document used to differentiate between levels of development in a specific skill performance or behavior. Rubrics are provided in this supplement for use as either a self-assessment tool to aid the student in behavior development or as an educator assessment tool to determine competence. Space is provided to record steps needed for further growth and improvement.

Performance is evaluated according to the following scale:

1 **Development Opportunity:** There is little or no evidence of competency; Assistance is needed; Performance includes multiple errors.

2 **Fundamental:** There is beginning evidence of competency; Task is completed alone; Performance includes few errors.

3 **Competent:** There is detailed and consistent evidence of competency; Task is completed alone; Performance includes rare errors.

4 **Strength:** There is detailed evidence of highly creative, inventive, mature presence of competency. Space is provided for comments to assist you in improving your performance and achieving a higher rating.

PERFORMANCE ASSESSED	1	2	3	4	IMPROVEMENT PLAN
Procedure					
1. Undraped the back.					
2. Standing at the client's side, applied lubricant to the back using light effleurage strokes.					
3. Applied effleurage from the iliac crest, up the back to the nape of the neck, over the shoulders, down the sides of the torso to the hips, and back to the starting point three to five times.					
4-5 Applied petrissage to the half of the client's back that is opposite you.					
6. Applied deep, alternate hand gliding strokes (shingles) to the far side of the client's body from the neck to the upper thigh and back up to the shoulder.					
7. Moved to the other side of the massage table.					
7a. Applied effleurage from the iliac crest, up the back to the nape of the neck, over the shoulders, down the sides of the torso to the hips, and back to the starting point three to five times.					
7b. Applied petrissage to the half of the client's back that is opposite you.					
7c. Applied deep, alternate-hand gliding strokes (shingles) to the far side of the client's body from the neck to the upper thigh and back up to the shoulder.					
8. Flexed the client's elbow and elevated the shoulder.					

PERFORMANCE ASSESSED	1	2	3	4	IMPROVEMENT PLAN
9. Applied kneading movements around the scapula.					
10. Applied friction and deep pressure along the vertebral border of the scapula.					
11. With the arm in the same position, lifted and rotated the shoulder.					
12a. Abducted the elbow and supported the arm just proximal to the elbow and swung the forearm back and forth to rotate the arm at the shoulder.					
12b. Replaced the arm on the table next to the client and moved to the other side of the table.					
13a. Flexed the client's other elbow and elevated the shoulder in order to apply kneading and friction movements around the scapula.					
13b. With the arm in the same position, lifted and rotated the shoulder.					
13c. Abducted the elbow and supported the arm just proximal to the elbow and swung the forearm back and forth to rotate the arm at the shoulder.					
13d. Replaced the arm on the table next to the client.					
14. Repeated the effleurage stroke to the entire back.					
15. Applied deep effleurage stroke from the midline to the side of the back (fan stroke), beginning on the upper back with consecutive strokes and moving down to the lower back.					
16. Applied wringing from the lower back to the nape of the neck and back down to the lower back.					
17. Applied deep, circular friction on the sacrospinalis muscles along the spine.					
18. Applied sacrospinalis vibration from the nape of the neck to the sacrum.					
19. Applied percussion (hacking) to the back (avoided the kidney area).					
20. Applied beating over the thicker muscles of the gluteals and back of legs. (optional)					
21. Applied cupping over the lungs. (optional)					
22. Applied light slapping over the entire back of the body.					
23–24. Applied a caring stroke from the head of the table.					
25. Placed one hand on the sacrum and the other at the base of the neck and applied a gentle rocking to complete the massage.					

Notes

Notes

Notes

Notes

Notes

Notes